DIGESTIVE DISEASES - RESEARCH AND CLINICAL DEVELOPMENTS

UNCOMMON GASTROINTESTINAL DISORDERS

DIAGNOSIS AND MANAGEMENT

Digestive Diseases - Research and Clinical Developments

Additional books in this series can be found on Nova's website under the Series tab.

Additional e-books in this series can be found on Nova's website under the e-book tab.

DIGESTIVE DISEASES - RESEARCH AND CLINICAL DEVELOPMENTS

UNCOMMON GASTROINTESTINAL DISORDERS

DIAGNOSIS AND MANAGEMENT

SACHIN B. INGLE
BABAN D. ADGAONKAR
CHITRA R. HINGE
AND
SALEHA SIDDIQUI

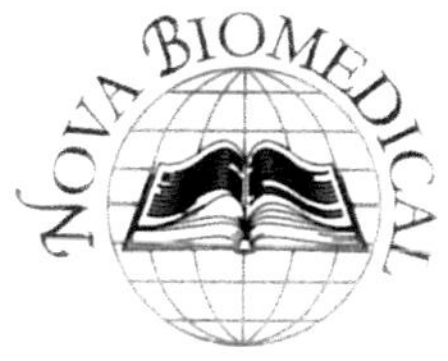

New York

NOTICE TO THE READER

The Publisher has taken reasonable care in the preparation of this book, but makes no expressed or implied warranty of any kind and assumes no responsibility for any errors or omissions. No liability is assumed for incidental or consequential damages in connection with or arising out of information contained in this book. The Publisher shall not be liable for any special, consequential, or exemplary damages resulting, in whole or in part, from the readers' use of, or reliance upon, this material. Any parts of this book based on government reports are so indicated and copyright is claimed for those parts to the extent applicable to compilations of such works.

Independent verification should be sought for any data, advice or recommendations contained in this book. In addition, no responsibility is assumed by the publisher for any injury and/or damage to persons or property arising from any methods, products, instructions, ideas or otherwise contained in this publication.

This publication is designed to provide accurate and authoritative information with regard to the subject matter covered herein. It is sold with the clear understanding that the Publisher is not engaged in rendering legal or any other professional services. If legal or any other expert assistance is required, the services of a competent person should be sought. FROM A DECLARATION OF PARTICIPANTS JOINTLY ADOPTED BY A COMMITTEE OF THE AMERICAN BAR ASSOCIATION AND A COMMITTEE OF PUBLISHERS.

Additional color graphics may be available in the e-book version of this book.

Library of Congress Cataloging-in-Publication Data

ISBN: 978-1-63482-005-9
Library of Congress Control Number: 2015932298

Published by Nova Science Publishers, Inc. † New York

Contents

Preface

Uncommon gastrointestinal diseases are the worrisome and challenging problem for the gastroenterologists and GI Pathologist. In this book, the authors present research in the study of the epidemiology, management and prevention of uncommon gastrointestinal diseases e.g., Isolated Gastroduodenal Crohn's Disease, Primary lymphangiectasis of intestine, Microscopic colitis, Eosinophilic gastroenteritis, Solitary rectal ulcer syndrome and Primary splenic epithelial cysts. This book is definitely useful to the Gastroenterologists and GI pathologists for diagnosis, treatment and prevention of these uncommon conditions.

Chapter 1 - Eosinophilic gastroenteritis (EGE) is a rare disorder characterized by eosinophilic infiltration of the bowel wall with various gastrointestinal manifestations. Till date, only 280 cases have been described in the literature. A high index of suspicion, by excluding other causes of peripheral eosinophilia, is a prerequisite for accurate diagnosis. EGE is an uncommon gastrointestinal disease affecting both children and adults. It was first described by Kaijser in 1937. Presentation may vary depending on location as well as depth and extent of bowel wall involvement and usually runs a chronic relapsing course. This condition can respond to low dose steroid therapy, thereby preventing grave complications like ascites and intestinal obstruction that might need surgical intervention. The natural history of EGE has not been well documented. Eosinophilic gastroenteritis is a chronic, waxing and waning condition. Mild and sporadic symptoms can be managed with reassurance and observation, whereas disabling gastrointestinal (GI) symptom flare-ups can often be controlled with oral corticosteroids. When the disease manifests in infancy and specific food sensitization can be identified, the likelihood of disease remission by late childhood is high. GI obstruction is the most common complication. Fatal outcomes are rare.

Chapter 2 - Microscopic colitis (MC) is characterized by chronic, watery, secretory diarrhea, with a normal or near normal gross appearance of the colonic mucosa. Biopsy is diagnostic and usually reveals either lymphocytic colitis or collagenous colitis. The symptoms of collagenous colitis appear most commonly in the sixth decade. Patients report watery, nonbloody diarrhea of a chronic, intermittent or chronic recurrent course. With collagenous colitis, the major microscopic characteristic is a thickened collagen layer beneath the colonic mucosa, and with lymphocytic colitis, an increased number of intraepithelial lymphocytes. Histological workup can confirm a diagnosis of MC and distinguish the two distinct histological forms, namely, collagenous and lymphocytic colitis. Presently, both forms are diagnosed and treated in the same way; thus, the description of the two forms is not of clinical value although this may change in the future. Since microscopic colitis was first described in 1976 and was only recently recognized as a common cause of diarrhea, many practicing physicians may not be aware of this entity. In this review, we outline the epidemiology, risk factors associated with MC, its etiopathogenesis, the approach to diagnosis and the management of these individuals.

Chapter 3 - Crohn's disease (CD) is a chronic idiopathic inflammatory disease of gastrointestinal tract characterized by segmental and transmural involvement of gastrointestinal tract. Ileocolonic and colonic/anorectal is a most common and account for 40% of cases and involvement of small intestine in about 30%. The stomach is rarely the sole or predominant site of CD. To date there are only a few documented case reports of adults with isolated gastric CD and no reports in the pediatric population. Isolated stomach involvement is a very unusual presentation accounting for less than 0.07% of all gastrointestinal CD. The diagnosis is difficult to establish in cases of atypical presentation as in isolated gastroduodenal disease. In the absence of any other source of disease and in the presence of nonspecific upper GI endoscopy and histological findings, serological testing can play a vital role in the diagnosis of atypical CD. Recent studies have suggested that perinuclear anti-neutrophil cytoplasmic antibody and anti-*Saccharomycescervisia* antibody may be used as additional diagnostic tools. The effectiveness of infliximab in isolated gastric CD is limited to only a few case reports of adult patients and the long-term outcome is unknown.

Chapter 4 - Primary idiopathic intestinal lymphangiectasia is an unusual disease featured by the presence of dilated lymphatic channels which are located in the mucosa, submucosa or subserosa leading to protein losing enteropathy. Most often affected were children who were generally diagnosed before their third year of life but this disease may be rarely seen in adults too. Bilateral pitting oedema of lower limb is the main clinical manifestation mimicking the systemic disease and posing a real diagnostic dilemma to the clinicians to differentiate it from other common systemic diseases like Congestive cardiac failure, Nephrotic Syndrome, Protein Energy Malnutrition, etc. Diagnosis can be made on capsule endoscopy which can localise the lesion but unable to take biopsy samples. Thus, recently double-balloon enteroscopy and biopsy in combination can be used as an effective diagnostic tool to hit the correct diagnosis. Patients respond dramatically to diets constituting of low long chain triglycerides and high protein content with supplements of medium chain triglyceride. Early diagnosis is important to prevent untoward complications related to disease or treatment for the sake of accurate pathological diagnosis.

Chapter 5 - Primary splenic epithelial cyst is an unusual event in everyday surgical practice with about 800 cases reported until date in the English literature. Splenic cysts may be parasitic or non-parasitic in origin. Nonparasitic cysts are either primary or secondary. Primary cysts are also called true, congenital, epidermoid or epithelial cysts. Primary splenic cysts account for 10% of all benign non-parasitic splenic cysts and are the most frequent type of splenic cysts in children. Usually, splenic cysts are asymptomatic and can be found incidentally during imaging techniques or on laprotomy. The symptoms are related to the size of cysts. When they assume large sizes, they may present with fullness in the left abdomen, local or referred pain, symptoms due to compression of adjacent structures (like nausea, vomiting, flatulence, diarrhea) or rarely thrombocytopenia, and occasionally complications such as infection, rupture and/or haemorrhage. The preoperative diagnosis of primary splenic cysts can be ascertained by ultrasonography (USG), computed tomography or magnetic resonance imaging, although the wide use of USG today has led to an increase in the incidence of splenic cysts by 1%. However, careful histopathological evaluation along with immunostaining for presence of epithelial lining is mandatory to arrive at the diagnosis. The treatment has changed drastically from total splenectomy in the past to splenic preservation methods recently.

Chapter 6 - Melanosis coli, also *pseudomelanosis coli*, is a disorder of pigmentation of the wall of the colon, often identified at the time of colonoscopy. It is benign, and may have no significant correlation with disease. The brown pigment is lipofuscin in macrophages, not melanin.

Chapter 1

Eosinophilic Gastroenteritis: An Unusual Type of Gastroenteritis

Introduction

Eosinophilic gastroenteritis is a rare disorder that can present with various gastrointestinal manifestations depending on the specific site and specific layer of the gastrointestinal tract involved. Majority of the cases involve stomach and proximal small bowel. The diagnostic criteria include demonstration of eosinophilic infiltration of bowel wall, lack of evidence of extra intestinal disease and exclusion of other causes of peripheral eosinophilia [1-4].

Eosinophilic gastroenteritis is characterized by the presence of abnormal gastrointestinal (GI) symptoms, most often abdominal pain, eosinophilic infiltration in one or more areas of the GI tract, defined as 50 or more eosinophils per high-power field, the absence of an identified cause of eosinophilia and the exclusion of eosinophilic involvement in organs other than the GI tract.

It can be classified into mucosal, muscular and serosal types based on the depth of involvement [5, 6]. The stomach is the organ most commonly affected, followed by small intestine and colon [7, 8]. The anatomical locations of eosinophilic infiltrates and the depth of GI involvement determine clinical symptoms. The therapeutic role of steroids and antihelminthic drugs in the treatment of eosinophilic gastroenteritis is not established. In a few cases, steroids have produced symptomatic improvement in controlling malabsorption syndrome [1, 9].

Epidemiology

Eosinophilic gastroenteritis occurs over a wide age range from infancy through the seventh decade, but most commonly between third to fifth decades of life [10, 11]. A slight male preponderance has been reported [12].

Although cases have been reported worldwide, the exact incidence of eosinophilic gastroenteritis is unclear. After first described by Kaijser [10], a little less than 300 cases have been reported in the literature. Kim et al. [2] reported 31 new cases of eosinophilic gastroenteritis in Seoul, Korea, between January 1970 and July 2003.

Venkataraman et al. [5] reported 7 cases of eosinophilic gastroenteritis over a 10-year period in India [5]. Chen et al. [3] reported 15 patients including 2 children, with eosinophilic gastroenteritis in 2003. In eosinophilic enteritis the morbidity is mainly due to combination of chronic nonspecific GI symptoms which include abdominal pain, nausea, vomiting, diarrhea, weight loss, and abdominal distension and more serious complications like intestinal obstruction and perforation [13, 14].

Pathophysiology

Eosinophilic gastroenteritis can involve any part of gastrointestinal tract from esophagus down to the rectum. The stomach and duodenum are the most common sites of involvement [1, 13-17]. The etiology and pathogenesis is not well understood. There is evidence to suggest that a hypersensitivity reaction may play a role. The clinical presentations of eosinophilic gastroenteritis vary according to the site and depth of eosinophilic intestinal infiltration. The presence of peripheral eosinophilia, abundant eosinophils in the gastrointestinal tract and dramatic response to steroids provide some support that the disease is mediated by a hypersensitivity reaction [1, 18]. Moreover, a study at Mayo clinic showed that 50% of patients with eosinophilic gastroenteritis give history of allergy such as asthma, rhinitis, drug allergy and eczema [1]. Peripheral blood eosinophilia and elevated serum immunoglobulin E (IgE) are usual but not universal. The damage to the gastrointestinal tract wall is caused by eosinophilic infiltration and degranulation [19]. Eosinophils are normally present in gastrointestinal mucosa as a part of host defense mechanism, though the finding in deeper tissue is almost always pathologic [20]. In eosinophilic gastroenteritis (EGE) cytokines interleukin (IL)-3, IL-5 and granulocyte macrophage colony stimulating factor may be responsible for the recruitment and activation of eosinophils and hence the pathogenesis. They have been observed immunohistochemically in diseased intestinal wall [21]. In addition eotaxin has been shown to have an integral role in regulating the homing of eosinophils into the lamina propria of stomach and small intestine [22]. Indeed, many patients have history of food allergy and other atopic conditions like eczema, asthma etc. In this allergic subtype of disease, it is thought that food allergens cross the intestinal mucosa and trigger an inflammatory response that includes mast cell degranulation and recruitment of eosinophils [23, 24].

Clinical Presentations

The clinical presentations of eosinophilic gastroenteritis vary according to the site and depth of inflammatory involvement of different layers of the intestinal wall. Approximately 80% have symptoms for several years [25]. Occasionally, the disease may manifest itself as an acute abdomen or bowel obstruction [13, 14]. Children and adolescents can present with growth retardation, failure to thrive, delayed puberty or amenorrhea. Adults have abdominal pain, diarrhea or dysphagia. Mucosal disease is the commonest variety that presents with features of protein losing enteropathy, bleeding or malabsorption. Failure to thrive and anaemia may also be present. Lower gastrointestinal bleeding may imply colonic involvement [1, 26, 27]. Involvement of muscle layer may cause bowel wall thickening and intestinal obstruction. Cramping and abdominal pain associated with nausea and vomiting occurs frequently. It can also present as an obstructing caecal mass or intussusception. The subserosal form, which is least common but can cause more morbidity, usually presents as eosinophilic ascites, which is usually an exudate, with abundant peripheral eosinophilia. Serosal and visceral peritoneal inflammation leads to leakage of fluids but has a more favourable response to corticosteroids. In literature features like cholangitis, pancreatitis [28], eosinophilic splenitis, acute appendicitis and giant refractory duodenal ulcer are also mentioned.

Diagnostic Evaluation

Four criteria are required for the diagnosis of eosinophilic gastroenteritis namely-presence of gastrointestinal symptoms, eosinophilic infiltration of gastrointestinal tract, exclusion of parasitic disease and absence of other systemic involvement. The presence of peripheral eosinophilia is not a universal phenomenon [1, 29].

A thorough evaluation of the patient is necessary, starting with laboratory evaluation.

After a detailed history and physical examination, a complete blood count plays an important role. Peripheral blood eosinophilia is found in 20%-80% of cases. Average count is 2000 eosinophils (eos)/μL in patients with mucosal layer involvement, 1000 eos/μL in patients with muscle layer involvement, and 8000 eos/μL in patients with serosal involvement. Iron-deficiency anemia may be evident on mean corpuscular volume. Serum albumin may be low, especially in patients with mucosal involvement.

Fecal protein loss can be assessed by measuring alpha1-antitrypsin in a 24-h feces collection. It is used to identify the inability to digest and absorb proteins in the GI tract. The normal value is 0-54 mg/dL. Patients with eosinophilic gastroenteritis have elevated alpha1-antitrypsin in their feces. Protein loss can also result in low levels of total immunoglobulins, but serum IgE could be elevated, which then strongly supports the diagnosis of eosinophilic gastroenteritis in conjunction with other findings. The erythrocyte sedimentation rate can be elevated in few cases.

Stool examination should be performed to rule out parasitic infestation. Mild-to-moderate steatorrhea is present in approximately 30% of patients. This can be measured by qualitative and quantitative stool tests. Skin prick tests help to identify sensitization to specific ingestant and/or inhalant allergens.

Computed tomography (CT) scan may show nodular and irregular thickening of the folds in the distal stomach and proximal small bowel, but these findings can also be present in other conditions like Crohn's disease and lymphoma. On ultrasonography ascitic fluid is usually detected in patients with serosal involvement.

Radiographic changes are variable, nonspecific, and/or absent in at least 40% of patients. Gastric folds can be enlarged, with or without nodular filling defects. In extensive disease strictures, ulceration or polypoid lesions may occur and valvulae conniventes may be thickened and flattened. In eosinophilic gastroenteritis involving the muscle layer, localized involvement of the antrum and pylorus may occur, causing narrowing of the distal antrum and gastric retention. The small intestine may be dilated, with an increase in the thickness of the mucosal folds. Prominent mucosal folds may be observed in the colon. Other tests like exploratory laparotomy may be indicated in patients with serosal eosinophilic gastroenteritis.

The endoscopic appearance is nonspecific. It includes erythematous, friable, nodular, and occasional ulcerative changes [3] (Figure 1). Sometimes diffuse inflammation results in complete loss of villi, involvement of multiple layers, submucosal oedema and fibrosis [30, 31]. When performing endoscopy, it is necessary to obtain at least 6 biopsy specimens from normal and abnormal areas of the bowel to exclude the possibility of sampling error. In patients with esophageal or colonic symptoms, additional biopsy specimens may be obtained from the relevant sites to aid the diagnosis.

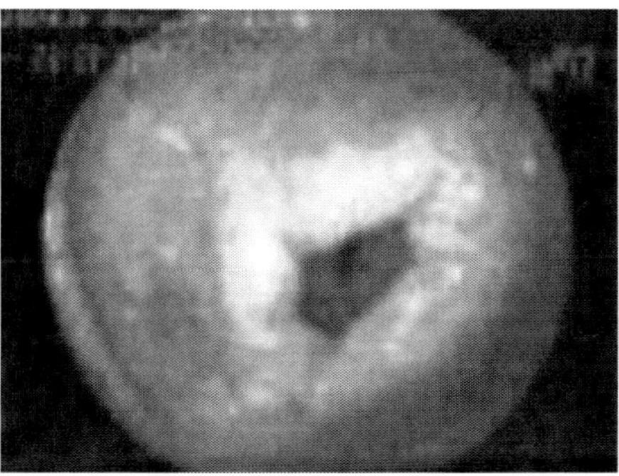

Figure 1. Endoscopy showing small superficial ulcers in stomach.

Patients with serosal disease present with ascites. Abdominal paracentesis demonstrates a sterile fluid with a high eosinophil count. Pleural effusion also may be present.

The diagnosis can be confirmed on histopathological examination of gastric and duodenal biopsies. The gross appearance of eosinophilic gastroenteritis upon endoscopy shows erythematous, friable, nodular, and often ulcerated mucosa. Microscopy demonstrates increased numbers of eosinophils (often > 50 eos per high-power field) in the lamina propria. Large numbers of eosinophils are often present in the muscularis and serosa (Figure 2). Localized eosinophilic infiltrates may cause crypt hyperplasia, epithelial cell necrosis, and villous atrophy. Diffuse enteritis with complete loss of villi, submucosal edema, infiltration of the GI wall, and fibrosis may be apparent. Mast cell infiltrates and hyperplastic mesenteric lymph nodes infiltrated with eosinophils may be present [1, 27, 31, 32]. Infiltration is often patchy, can be missed and laparoscopic full thickness biopsy may be required.

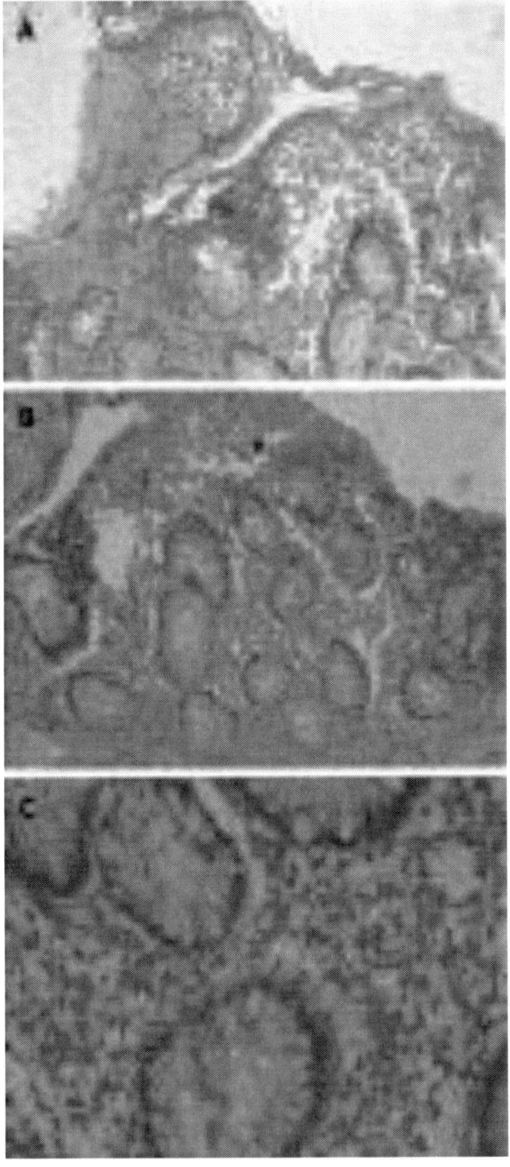

Figure 2. Large numbers of eosinophils are often present in the muscularis and serosa. A, B: Showing dense eosinophilic infiltrates in the lamina propria and mucosa (× 10); C: Showing dense eosinophilic infiltrates in the lamina propria and mucosa.

Histologic analysis of the small intestine reveals increased deposition of extracellular major basic proteins and eosinophilic cationic proteins.

Radio isotope scan using technetium (^{99m}Tc) exametazime-labeled leukocyte single-photon emission CT may be useful in assessing the extent of disease and response to treatment but has little value in diagnosis, as the scan does not help differentiating EGE from other causes of inflammation [33, 34].

When eosinophilic gastroenteritis is observed in association with eosinophilic infiltration of other organ systems, the diagnosis of idiopathic hypereosinophilic syndrome should be considered [35].

Differential Diagnosis

The main differential diagnoses are: (1) eosinophilic esophagitis; (2) eosinophilic ascites; (3) coeliac disease; (4) protein losing enteropathy from intolerance to cow milk protein; (5) infantile formula protein intolerance; and (6) idiopathic hypereosinophilic syndrome.

A diagnosis of idiopathic hypereosinophilic syndrome can be ruled out when there is absence of eosinophilic infiltration in all other organs except the bowel [35].

In celiac disease, biopsy of small bowel shows blunting of villi, crypt hyperplasia, and predominantly lymphocyte infiltration of crypts. Coeliac disease is caused by a reaction to gliadin, a prolamin (glutenprotein) found in wheat, and similar proteins found in other grains [36].

In eosinophilic esophagitis only the eosophagus is involved and not the whole bowel. A minimum of 15 eosinophils per high power field is required to make the diagnosis. Typically, eosinophils can be found in superficial clusters near the surface of the epithelium. An expansion of the basal layer is also seen in response to the inflammatory damage to the epithelium. At the time of endoscopy, ridges or furrows may be seen in the esophageal mucosa. Presence of white exudates in esophagus is also suggestive of the diagnosis [37, 38].

Treatment

The role of steroids and antihelminthic drugs is not well established. However, in a few cases, steroids have been reported to produce symptomatic improvement in controlling diarrhea and protein losing enteropathy [9].

Corticosteroids are the mainstay of therapy with a 90% response rate in some studies (Figure 3). Appropriate duration of steroid treatment is unknown and relapse often necessitates long term treatment. Various steroid sparing agents, e.g., sodium cromoglycate (a stabilizer of mast cell membranes), ketotifen (an antihistamine), and montelukast (a selective, competitive leukotriene receptor antagonist) have been proposed, centering around an allergic hypothesis, with mixed results [24, 39, 40].

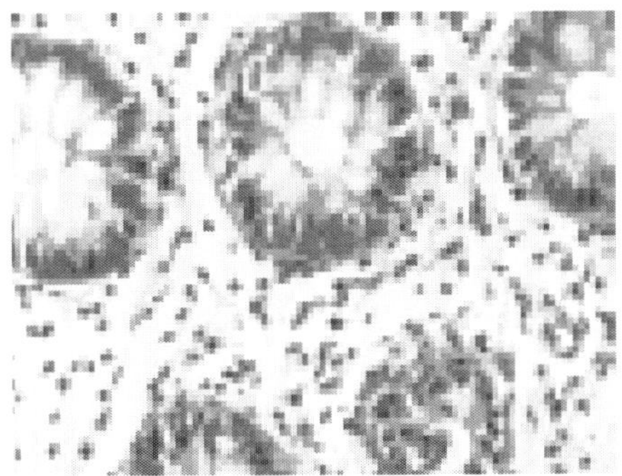

Figure 3. Post treatment (low dose steroid) biopsy showing resolution of disease.

Corticosteroids

Fluticasone inhaled (Flovent): Decreases recruitment of inflammatory cells including eosinophils and decreases the release of eotaxins and other inflammatory mediators. Dosage required is higher than that used in asthma.

Prednisolone (AK-Pred, Delta-Cortef): Decreases inflammation by suppressing migration of polymorphonuclear leukocytes and reducing capillary permeability. Equivalent dosages of prednisone or methyl-prednisolone may be used.

Budesonide (Pulmicort Respule) oral viscous suspension: Decreases inflammation, reduces capillary permeability [6].

Mast Cell Stabilizers

Cromolyn (Intal, Gastrocrom): Inhibits release of histamine, leukotrienes, and other mediators from sensitized mast cells. It also inhibits the influx of neutrophils, as well as the formation of the active form of NADPH oxidase, which in turn prevents tissue damage caused by oxygen radicals.

Leukotriene Receptor Antagonists

Prevent or reverse some of the pathologic features associated with the inflammatory process mediated by leukotrienes C4, D4 and E4. Successful treatment of eosinophilic gastroenteritis has been reported in few cases, mainly with Montelukast (Singulair) which is a potent and selective antagonist of leukotriene D4 at the cysteinyl leukotriene receptor, CysLT1 [41].

Role of surgical Care

Surgery is avoided, except when it is necessary to relieve persistent pyloric or small bowel obstruction. Most patients respond to conservative measures and oral glucocorticosteroids. Recurrence is possible, even after surgical excision.

Prognosis

The natural history of EGE has not been well documented. Eosinophilic gastroenteritis is a chronic, waxing and waning condition. Mild and sporadic symptoms can be managed with reassurance and observation, whereas disabling GI symptom flare-ups can often be controlled with oral corticosteroids. When the disease manifests in infancy and specific food sensitization can be identified, the likelihood of disease remission by late childhood is high. GI obstruction is the most common complication. Fatal outcomes are rare.

Preventive and Diet Therapy

The strong association of eosinophilic gastroenteritis with food allergies has prompted the use of restrictive or elemental diets. Initially, a trial elimination diet that excludes milk, eggs, wheat and/or gluten, soy, and beef may be helpful. Skin testing can identify food hypersensitivity. If a prohibitive number of food reactions are found, an amino-acid-based diet or elemental diet may be considered. Educate patients to avoid foods that they cannot tolerate and to seek medical care when needed.

Differential Diagnosis

The main differential diagnoses are: (1) eosinophilic esophagitis; (2) eosinophilic ascites; (3) coeliac disease; (4) protein losing enteropathy from intolerance to cow milk protein; (5) infantile formula protein intolerance; and (6) idiopathic hypereosinophilic syndrome.

A diagnosis of idiopathic hypereosinophilic syndrome can be ruled out when there is absence of eosinophilic infiltration in all other organs except the bowel [35].

In celiac disease, biopsy of small bowel shows blunting of villi, crypt hyperplasia, and predominantly lymphocyte infiltration of crypts. Coeliac disease is caused by a reaction to gliadin, a prolamin (glutenprotein) found in wheat, and similar proteins found in other grains [36].

In eosinophilic esophagitis only the eosophagus is involved and not the whole bowel. A minimum of 15 eosinophils per high power field is required to make the diagnosis. Typically, eosinophils can be found in superficial clusters near the surface of the epithelium. An expansion of the basal layer is also seen in response to the inflammatory damage to the epithelium. At the time of endoscopy, ridges or furrows may be seen in the esophageal mucosa. Presence of white exudates in esophagus is also suggestive of the diagnosis [37, 38].

References

[1] Ingle SB, Patle YG, Murdeshwar HG, Pujari GP. A case of early eosinophilic gastroenteritis with dramatic response to steroids. *J Crohns Colitis*. 2011;5:71–72. [PubMed]

[2] Kim NI, Jo YJ, Song MH, Kim SH, Kim TH, Park YS, Eom WY, Kim SW. Clinical features of eosinophilic gastroenteritis. *Korean J Gastroenterol. 2004*;44:217–223. [PubMed]

[3] Chen MJ, Chu CH, Lin SC, Shih SC, Wang TE. Eosinophilic gastroenteritis: clinical experience with 15 patients. *World J Gastroenterol.* 2003;9:2813–2816. [PubMed]

[4] Hsu YQ, Lo CY. A case of eosinophilic gastroenteritis. *Hong Kong Med J.* 1998;4:226–228. [PubMed]

[5] Venkataraman S, Ramakrishna BS, Mathan M, Chacko A, Chandy G, Kurian G, Mathan VI. Eosinophilic gastroenteritis--an Indian experience. *Indian J Gastroenterol.* 1998;17:148–149. [PubMed]

[6] Aceves SS, Bastian JF, Newbury RO, Dohil R. Oral viscous budesonide: a potential new therapy for eosinophilic esophagitis in children. *Am J Gastroenterol.* 2007;102:2271–2279; quiz 2280. [PubMed]

[7] Chehade M, Magid MS, Mofidi S, Nowak-Wegrzyn A, Sampson HA, Sicherer SH. Allergic eosinophilic gastroenteritis with protein-losing enteropathy: intestinal pathology, clinical course, and long-term follow-up. *J Pediatr Gastroenterol Nutr.* 2006;42:516–521. [PubMed]

[8] De Angelis P, Morino G, Pane A, Torroni F, Francalanci P, Sabbi T, Foschia F, Caldaro T, di Abriola GF, Dall'Oglio L. Eosinophilic esophagitis: management and pharmacotherapy. *Expert Opin Pharmacother.* 2008;9:731–740. [PubMed]

[9] Sharma S, Singh M, Naik S, Kumar S, Varshney S. Case report of eosinophilic gastroenteritis. *Bmbay Hospital Journal.* 2004:46. Available from: http://www.bhj.org.in/journal/2004_4603_july/july_2004/htm/case_reports_eosonophilic.htm.

[10] Kaijser R. Zur Kenntnis der allergischen Affektionen des Verdauugskanals vom Standpunkt des Chirurgen aus. *Arch Klin Chir.* 1937;188:36–64. Available from: http://ci.nii.ac.jp/naid/10010523250/

[11] Klein NC, Hargrove RL, Sleisenger MH, Jeffries GH. Eosinophilic gastroenteritis. *Medicine (Baltimore.)* 1970;49:299–319. [PubMed]

[12] Guandalini S. *Essential pediatric gastroenterology, hepatology and nutrition.* New York: McGraw Hill; 2004. p. 210.

[13] Shweiki E, West JC, Klena JW, Kelley SE, Colley AT, Bross RJ, Tyler WB. Eosinophilic gastroenteritis presenting as an obstructing cecal mass--a case report and review of the literature. *Am J Gastroenterol.* 1999;94:3644–3645. [PubMed]

[14] Tran D, Salloum L, Tshibaka C, Moser R. Eosinophilic gastroenteritis mimicking acute appendicitis. *Am Surg.* 2000;66:990–992. [PubMed]

[15] Schulze K, Mitros FA. Eosinophilic gastroenteritis involving the ileocecal area. *Dis Colon Rectum.* 1979;22:47–50. [PubMed]

[16] Chisholm JC, Martin HI. Eosinophilic gastroenteritis with rectal involvement: case report and a review of literature. *J Natl Med Assoc.* 1981;73:749–753. [PMC free article] [PubMed]

[17] Moore D, Lichtman S, Lentz J, Stringer D, Sherman P. Eosinophilic gastroenteritis presenting in an adolescent with isolated colonic involvement. Gut. 1986;27:1219–1222. [PMC free article] [PubMed]

[18] Dobbins JW, Sheahan DG, Behar J. Eosinophilic gastroenteritis with esophageal involvement. *Gastroenterology.* 1977;72:1312–1316. [PubMed]

[19] Talley NJ, Shorter RG, Phillips SF, Zinsmeister AR. Eosinophilic gastroenteritis: a clinicopathological study of patients with disease of the mucosa, muscle layer, and subserosal tissues. *Gut.* 1990;31:54–58. [PMC free article] [PubMed]

[20] Tan AC, Kruimel JW, Naber TH. Eosinophilic gastroenteritis treated with non-enteric-coated budesonide tablets. *Eur J Gastroenterol Hepatol.* 2001;13:425–427. [PubMed]

[21] Blackshaw AJ, Levison DA. Eosinophilic infiltrates of the gastrointestinal tract. *J Clin Pathol.* 1986;39:1–7. [PMC free article] [PubMed]

[22] Desreumaux P, Bloget F, Seguy D, Capron M, Cortot A, Colombel JF, Janin A. Interleukin 3, granulocyte-macrophage colony-stimulating factor, and interleukin 5 in eosinophilic gastroenteritis. *Gastroenterology.* 1996;110:768–774. [PubMed]

[23] Mishra A, Hogan SP, Brandt EB, Rothenberg ME. An etiological role for aeroallergens and eosinophils in experimental esophagitis. *J Clin Invest.* 2001;107:83–90. [PMC free article] [PubMed]

[24] Pérez-Millán A, Martín-Lorente JL, López-Morante A, Yuguero L, Sáez-Royuela F. Subserosal eosinophilic gastroenteritis treated efficaciously with sodium cromoglycate. *Dig Dis Sci.* 1997;42:342–344. [PubMed]

[25] Christopher V, Thompson MH, Hughes S. Eosinophilic gastroenteritis mimicking pancreatic cancer. *Postgrad Med J.* 2002;78:498–499. [PMC free article] [PubMed]

[26] Baig MA, Qadir A, Rasheed J. A review of eosinophilic gastroenteritis. J Natl Med Assoc. 2006;98:1616–1619. [PMC free article] [PubMed]

[27] Lee CM, Changchien CS, Chen PC, Lin DY, Sheen IS, Wang CS, Tai DI, Sheen-Chen SM, Chen WJ, Wu CS. Eosinophilic gastroenteritis: 10 years experience. *Am J Gastroenterol.* 1993;88:70–74. [PubMed]

[28] Lyngbaek S, Adamsen S, Aru A, Bergenfeldt M. Recurrent acute pancreatitis due to eosinophilic gastroenteritis. Case report and literature review. *JOP.* 2006;7:211–217. [PubMed]

[29] Kamal MF, Shaker K, Jaser N, Leimoon BA. Eosinophilic gastroenteritis with no peripheral eosinophilia. *Ann Chir Gynaecol.* 1985;74:98–100. [PubMed]

[30] Johnstone JM, Morson BC. Eosinophilic gastroenteritis. *Histopathology.* 1978;2:335–348. [PubMed]

[31] Katz AJ, Goldman H, Grand RJ. Gastric mucosal biopsy in eosinophilic (allergic) gastroenteritis. *Gastroenterology.* 1977;73:705–709. [PubMed]

[32] Talley N. Eosinophilic Gastroenteritis. In: Feldman M, Scharschmidt BF, Sleisenger M, Zorab R, edtidors , et al., editors. *Sleisenger and Fordtran's Gastrointestinal and Liver Disease: Pathophysiology/Diagnosis/Management.* 6th ed. Philadelphia: WB Saunders; 1998. pp. 1679–1686.

[33] Lee KJ, Hahm KB, Kim YS, Kim JH, Cho SW, Jie H, Park CH, Yim H. The usefulness of Tc-99m HMPAO labeled WBC SPECT in eosinophilic gastroenteritis. *Clin Nucl Med.* 1997;22:536–541. [PubMed]

[34] Imai E, Kaminaga T, Kawasugi K, Yokokawa T, Furui S. The usefulness of 99mTc-hexamethylpropyleneamineoxime white blood cell scintigraphy in a patient with eosinophilic gastroenteritis. *Ann Nucl Med.* 2003;17:601–603. [PubMed]

[35] Matsushita M, Hajiro K, Morita Y, Takakuwa H, Suzaki T. Eosinophilic gastroenteritis involving the entire digestive tract. *Am J Gastroenterol.* 1995;90:1868–1870. [PubMed]

[36] Di Sabatino A, Corazza GR. Coeliac disease. *Lancet.* 2009;373:1480–1493. [PubMed]

[37] Zimmerman SL, Levine MS, Rubesin SE, Mitre MC, Furth EE, Laufer I, Katzka DA. Idiopathic eosinophilic esophagitis in adults: the ringed esophagus. *Radiology.* 2005;236:159–165. [PubMed]

[38] Samadi F, Levine MS, Rubesin SE, Katzka DA, Laufer I. Feline esophagus and gastroesophageal reflux. *AJR Am J Roentgenol.* 2010;194:972–976. [PubMed]

[39] Barbie DA, Mangi AA, Lauwers GY. Eosinophilic gastroenteritis associated with systemic lupus erythematosus. *J Clin Gastroenterol.* 2004;38:883–886. [PubMed]

[40] Moots RJ, Prouse P, Gumpel JM. Near fatal eosinophilic gastroenteritis responding to oral sodium chromoglycate. *Gut.* 1988;29:1282–1285. [PMC free article] [PubMed]

[41] Neustrom MR, Friesen C. Treatment of eosinophilic gastroenteritis with montelukast. *J Allergy Clin Immunol.* 1999;104:506. [PubMed]

Chapter 2

Primary Intestinal Lymphangiectasia

Abstract

Primary idiopathic intestinal lymphangiectasia is an unusual disease featured by the presence of dilated lymphatic channels which are located in the mucosa, submucosa or subserosa leading to protein loosing enteropathy. Most often affected were children and generally diagnosed before third year of life but may be rarely seen in adults too. Bilateral pitting oedema of lower limb is the main clinical manifestation mimicking the systemic disease and posing a real diagnostic dilemma to the clinicians to differentiate it from other common systemic diseases like Congestive cardiac failure, Nephrotic Syndrome, Protein Energy Malnutrition, etc. Diagnosis can be made on capsule endoscopy which can localize the lesion but unable to take biopsy samples. Thus, recently double-balloon enteroscopy and biopsy in combination can be used as an effective diagnostic tool to hit the correct diagnosis. Patients respond dramatically to diet constituting low long chain triglycerides and high protein content with supplements of medium chain triglyceride. So early diagnosis is important to prevent untoward complications related to disease or treatment for the sake of accurate pathological diagnosis.

Introduction

Primary Intestinal lymphangiectasia (PIL) was originally described in 1961 by Waldmann et al. [1]. It is an unusual cause of protein losing enteropathy either due to congenital malformation or obstruction of lymphatics of intestine [2]. Lymphangectasia is characterised by dilated and proliferating lymphatic channels located in mucosa, submucosa or subserosa leading to protein loosing enteropathy and loss of lymph into gut resulting in to hypoproteinemia, hypogammaglobulinemia, hypoalbuminemia and lymphopenia [3-5]. Peripheral oedema usually symmetrical (lower limb oedema) is the main clinical feature posing a real diagnostic dilemma to the clinicians to differentiate it from other common conditions like congestive cardiac failure, nephrotic syndrome, protein energy malnutrition, etc. [3]. Other symptoms are ascites, pleural effusion, weight loss and abdominal pain, diarrhoea with increased faecal loss of protein and fat with increased serum levels of α1-antitrypsin [2, 5]. Diagnosis is defined by endoscopic evaluation and confirmed on histopathological evaluation of biopsy of small intestine [1]. Now a day double balloon endoscopy and biopsy is the mainstay to arrive at correct diagnosis.

Epidemology

The worldwide incidence and prevalence of PIL is not known [2, 6]. After 1961, as per available literature less than 200 cases were reported [7, 8]. Very few familial forms are reported [1, 2, 9]. There is no specific predilection for sex and race [6]. Most commonly, it has been seen in children and majority of the cases were diagnosed at or before 3 years of age but can be seen in adults also [5, 6].

Pathophysiology

Waldmann's disease is also called as exudative enteropathy. The pathogenesis is not clear. The proposed hypothetical theories for pathogenesis are:

Lymphatic Obstruction Theory

The basic cause for protein loss in PIL is poorly understood although lymphatic channel malformation/lymphatic hypoplasia leads to obstruction in lymph flow with resultant increase in intraluminal pressure in lymphatic channels [6, 10, 11]. This, increased intraluminal pressure will cause dilatation of the submucosal, subserosal lymphatic vessels in the intestine finally leading to the rupture of the cystically dilated channels and leading to discharge of the lymph into the bowel lumen [6, 12]. Thus, net result is hypoalbuminemia, hypogammaglobinemia and lymphopenia.

Genetic Theory

There are mutations in genes that regulate the process of lymphogenesis [5]. Multiple genes, e.g., vascular endothelial growth factor receptor 3, prospero-related homeobox-transcriptional factor, forkhead transcriptional factor and *SOX18* play vital role in lymphogenesis [13]. Mutation of the *CCBE1* gene has been identified as a cause of intestinal lymphangiectasia in Hennekam syndrome.

Clinical Presenation

Age-PIL is mainly seen in paediatric age group (usually before 3 years of age) and young adults but may be diagnosed in adults too [2, 14-16].

Oedema is the main clinical manifestation. The patient may present with ascites, pleural effusion and pericarditis. Other symptoms are lymphedema, abdominal pain, fatigue, moderate diarrhoea, weight loss and deficiency of fat soluble vitamins may also be present.

Oedema is of pitting type and usually symmetrical in distribution involving lower limb. Sometimes severe oedema involving face, scrotum or vagina [5].

Rarely lymphedema have been described which is elicited by "stemmer's sign" and it is difficult to differentiate from other systemic causes of oedema [2, 5]. Sonographic evidence of fetal ascites had also been reported [2, 5, 17].

Non-specific clinical features such as fatigue, nausea, vomiting, abdominal pain, weight loss, failure to thrive, moderate diarrhoea with faecal loss of fat along with increased faecal loss of protein, leading to rise in alfa-1-antitrypsin levels and there is deficiency of fat soluble vitamins [5, 18].

Hypocalcemia-patients can also develop hypocalcemia and tetany due to vitamin D deficiency [2, 6, 19]. A case of digital clubbing in PIL was reported [20]. Osteomalacia and osteoporosis associated with PIL was reported [21].

Rare Associations-An association of PIL with celiac sprue was described [5, 22]. PIL has been reported as a rare cause of lower gastrointestinal bleeding. In addition iron deficiency may occur [5, 18]. Recently proved association with angiodysplasia leading to occult blood loss in PIL [5, 23, 24].

A case of intestinal lymphangiectasia presenting as abdominal mass was reported [2, 5, 25]. Recurrent haemolytic uraemic syndrome has been described in association with intestinal lymphangiectasia [2, 26]. Patients with PIL are prone to develop infections due to lymphopenia and hypogammaglobulinemia [18, 27].

Only two cases of disseminated cryptococcal meningitis and osteomyelitis in-patient with lymphangectasia have been reported in the literature so far [28-30]. Recently another case of cryptococcal meningitis as primary manifestation in a patient with intestinal lymphangiectasia has been reported [30]. Lymphoma may complicate the long term outcome of PIL patients [5, 31].

PIL may exist as a part of a genetic syndromes, i.e., Noonan, Von Recklinghausen, Hennekam and Yellow nail syndrome [2, 5, 14]. Finally, an association with autoimmune poly glandular disease type 1 has been described [5, 32, 33]. Recently a case of intestinal lymphangiectasia in a patient with infantile systemic hyalinosis syndrome has been reported [34].

Diagnostic Evaluation

Now days, diagnosis of Intestinal lymphangiectasia is based on characteristic findings during a double-balloon enteroscopy with further confirmation by histopathological examination of corresponding biopsy specimens [6, 35]. To confirm the primary nature of waldmanns disease we must first exclude the secondary causes of intestinal lymphangiectasia [6].

Capsule Endoscopy

Capsule endoscopy provides complete examination of small bowel mucosa thus can evaluate the extent of lymphangiectasia [36, 37]. However, the drawback of capsular endoscopy is the inability to obtain biopsies. So recently double balloon enteroscopy is evolved.

Double Balloon Enteroscopy

In view of the drawback of capsular endoscopy, its inability to obtain biopsies, double balloon enteroscopy was evolved which allowed obtaining biopsies from lesions detected by capsular endoscopy [35, 36].

Endoscopy reveals scattered white spots, which have been described as a characteristic snowflake appearance, (Figure 1) overlying the small intestinal mucosa [4, 38].

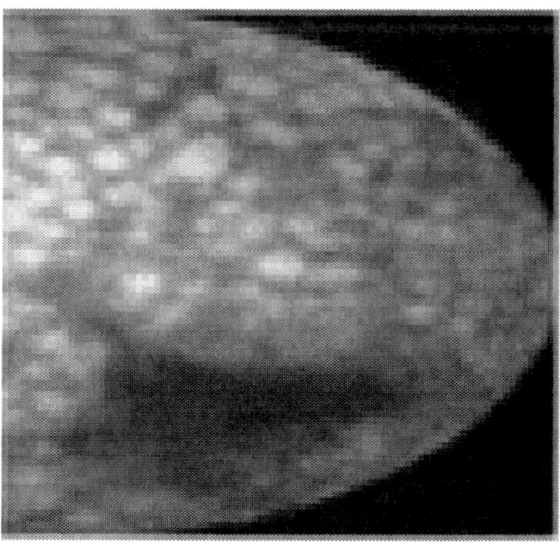

Figure 1. Snow flake appearance.

On Endoscopy

Histopathological examination of biopsies shows dilated lymphatic vessels in mucosa, submucosa and serosa with polyclonal plasma cells confirming the intestinal lymphangiectasia (Figure2).

Although various methods are available to investigate PIL, careful histopathological examination of biopsies is must to confirm the diagnosis. Various methods to investigate PIL are ^{99}Tc-HSA, 24 h stool alfa-1-antitrypsin clearances, lymphoscintigraphy, ultrasonography (USG), computed tomography (CT) scan, magnetic resonance imaging (MRI).

^{99}Technetium-labelled scintigraphy is useful to arrive at the diagnosis of PIL. Due to high cost and infectious risk, it has replaced with alfa-1-antitrypsin method [2, 39].

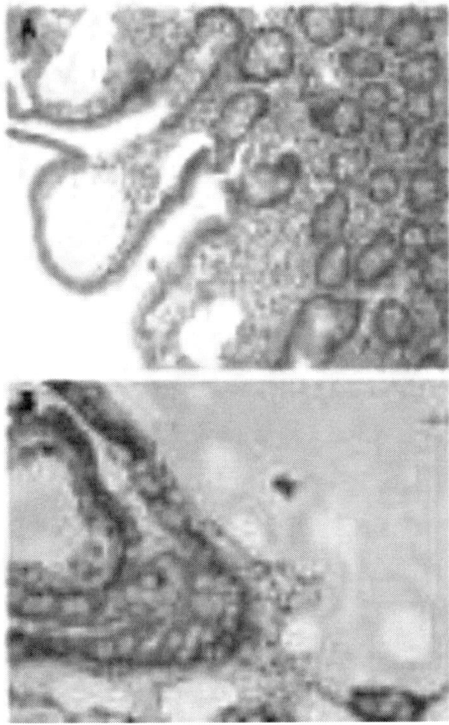

Figure 2. Histopathological examination of biopsies. A: Dilated lymphatics in mucosa and submucosa; B: 40 ×; showing dilated lymphatic channels filled with lymph.

Lymphoscintigraphy identifies abnormality in lymphatic tree but at present is not a routine method for PIL diagnosis [2, 40, 41].

On radiographic barium studies, thickened irregular mucosal fold with tiny nodules representing dilated lymphatic suggest the intestinal lymphangiectasia [42].

Non-Invasive Modalities

Imaging with USG/CT scan has shown diffuse thickening of small bowel wall because of engorgement of villi that contain the dilated lymphatic channels [5, 43]. CT scan may show "halo sign". A halo sign that consist of thickened, low-attenuation inner ring representing dilated lymphatics and higher attenuation outer ring, which consist of muscularis propria and serosa [43-45]. Nonenhanced, fluid-sensitive MRI may show bright signal intensity, which corresponds to lymphangiectasia in the mucosa [42, 44].

Other Laboratory Investigations

PIL is associated with many laboratory findings which include decreased albumin and total protein levels [2, 5, 45]. In Addition diminished immunoglobulins IgG, IgA and IgM suggesting B cell depletion and reduced numbers of $CD4^+$ cells as naive $CD45RA^+$ lymphocytes and $CD45RO^+CD8^+$T cells reflecting T-cell depletion seen [2, 5, 46, 47].

Finally, a recent report indicates there is failure of compensatory mechanism of production of T lymphocytes by the thymus to overcome the enteric loss of T lymphocytes leading to lymphopenia associated with lymphangiectasia [5, 48].

Differential Diagnosis

The differential diagnosis of PIL is large and involves many conditions producing protein-losinggastroenteropathy. Much closer differential are those, which involve protein loss associated with impaired intestinal lymphatic drainage. Such conditions include cardiac causes like congestive cardiac failure, constrictive pericarditis and cardiomyopathy [49-52]. Surgical repair of complex congenital heart disease (such as the Fontan procedure for a functional single ventricle), other conditions like lymphenteric fistula [10, 53], Whipple's disease [54], Crohn's disease [55], sarcoidosis [56], human immunodeficiency virus-related enteropathy [57], intestinal tuberculosis [58], radiation and/or chemotherapy with retroperitoneal fibrosis [59] and portal hypertension or hepatic venous outflow obstruction after liver transplantation and in congenital hepatic fibrosis due to phosphomannose isomerase deficiency [60].

Treatment

The principal treatment for PIL is diet rich in protein, low in fat with supplementation of medium chain triglyceride. Medium chain triglyceride is directly absorbed in portal venous circulation by passing the intestinal lymphatics, thus provides the energy and lessens lacteal engorgement and lymph loss.

A low fat diet reduces lymphatic flow and pressure preventing the lacteal dilation and lymph leakage resulting from their rupture. In some, reversal of clinical and biochemical changes has been seen with this dietary modification. In most patients, dietary treatment is permanently needed. This is found to be more effective in children than adults. In some cases, total parenteral nutrition is needed. Supportive therapy includes albumin infusion and paracentesis.

In patients, not responding to such therapy other options may be used after or in combination with dietary modification. These are octreotide, antiplasmin, tranexemic acid, vitamin D supplementation and surgical resection of segmental or localised intestinal lymphangiectasia [8, 11, 61].

To conclude PIL is an idiopathic protein loosing enteropathy either due to genetic defect or due to lymphatic obstruction. Careful endoscopic examination and meticulous histopathological evaluation is mandatory to arrive at correct pathological diagnosis to decide the proper treatment plan. One should keep in mind this rare condition as a differential diagnosis of oedema.

References

[1] Waldmann TA, Steinfeld JL, Dutcher TF, Davidson JD, Gordon RS. The role of the gastrointestinal system in "idiopathic hypoproteinemia" *Gastroenterology*. 1961;41:197–207. [PubMed]

[2] Vignes S, Bellanger J. Primary intestinal lymphangiectasia (Waldmann's disease) *Orphanet J Rare Dis*. 2008;3:5. [PMC free article] [PubMed]

[3] Katoch P, Bhardwaj S. Lymphangiectasia of small intestine presenting as intussusception. *Indian J Pathol Microbiol*. 2008;51:411–412. [PubMed]

[4] Abramowsky C, Hupertz V, Kilbridge P, Czinn S. Intestinal lymphangiectasia in children: a study of upper gastrointestinal endoscopic biopsies. *Pediatr Pathol*. 1989;9:289–297. [PubMed]

[5] Freeman HJ, Nimmo M. Intestinal lymphangiectasia in adults. *World J Gastrointest Oncol.* 2011;3:19–23. [PMC free article] [PubMed]

[6] Lai Y, Yu T, Qiao XY, Zhao LN, Chen QK. Primary intestinal lymphangiectasia diagnosed by double-balloon enteroscopy and treated by medium-chain triglycerides: a case report. *J Med Case Rep.* 2013;7:19. [PMC free article] [PubMed]

[7] Lee J, Kong MS. Primary intestinal lymphangiectasia diagnosed by endoscopy following the intake of a high-fat meal. *Eur J Pediatr.* 2008;167:237–239. [PubMed]

[8] Wen J, Tang Q, Wu J, Wang Y, Cai W. Primary intestinal lymphangiectasia: four case reports and a review of the literature. *Dig Dis Sci.* 2010;55:3466–3472. [PubMed]

[9] Le Bougeant P, Delbrel X, Grenouillet M, Leou S, Djossou F, Beylot J, Lebras M, Longy-Boursier M. Familial Waldmann's disease. *Ann Med Interne* (Paris) 2000;151:511–512. [PubMed]

[10] Mistilis SP, Skyring AP, Stephen DD. Intestinal lymphangiectasia mechanism of enteric loss of plasma-protein and fat. *Lancet.* 1965;1:77–79. [PubMed]

[11] Jeffries GH, Chapman A, Sleisenger MH. Low-fat diet in intestinal lymphangiectasia. its effect on albumin metabolism. *N Engl J Med.* 1964;270:761–766. [PubMed]

[12] Toskes P. Gastrointestinal diseases: malabsorption. In Cecil Textbook of Medicine. 18th edition. Wyngaarden J, Smith L (eds) Philadelphia: *WB Saunders;* 1988. pp. 732–745.

[13] Hokari R, Kitagawa N, Watanabe C, Komoto S, Kurihara C, Okada Y, Kawaguchi A, Nagao S, Hibi T, Miura S. Changes in regulatory molecules forlymphangiogenesis in intestinal lymphangiectasia with enteric protein loss. *J Gastroenterol Hepatol.* 2008;23:e88–95. [PubMed]

[14] Al Sinani S, Rawahi YA, Abdoon H. Octreotide in Hennekam syndrome-associated intestinal lymphangiectasia. *World J Gastroenterol.* 2012;18:6333–6337. [PMC free article] [PubMed]

[15] Boursier V, Vignes S. [Limb lymphedema as a first manifestation of primary intestinal lymphangiectasia (Waldmann's disease)] *J Mal Vasc.* 2004;29:103–106. [PubMed]

[16] Tift WL, Lloyd JK. Intestinal lymphangiectasia. Long-term results with MCT diet. *Arch Dis Child.* 1975;50:269–276. [PMC free article] [PubMed]

[17] Schmider A, Henrich W, Reles A, Vogel M, Dudenhausen JW. Isolated fetal ascites caused by primary lymphangiectasia: a case report. *Am J Obstet Gynecol.* 2001;184:227–228. [PubMed]

[18] Xinias I, Mavroudi A, Sapountzi E, Thomaidou A, Fotoulaki M, Kalambakas A, Karypidou E, Kollios K, Pardalos G, Imvrios G. Primary intestinal lymphangiectasia: is it always bad? Two cases with different outcome. *Case Rep Gastroenterol.* 2013;7:153–163. [PMC free article] [PubMed]

[19] Lu YY, Wu JF, Ni YH, Peng SS, Shun CT, Chang MH. Hypocalcemia and tetany caused by vitamin D deficiency in a child with intestinal lymphangiectasia. *J Formos Med Assoc.* 2009;108:814–818. [PubMed]

[20] Wiedermann CJ, Kob M, Benvenuti S, Carella R, Lucchin L, Piazzi L, Chilovi F, Mazzoleni G. Digital clubbing in primary intestinal lymphangiectasia: a case report. *Wien Med Wochenschr.* 2010;160:431–436. [PubMed]

[21] Li XP, Shen WB, Long MQ, Meng XW, Lian XL, Yu M. Osteomalacia and osteoporosis associated with primary intestinal lymphangiectasis. *Chin Med J* (Engl) 2012;125:1836–1838. [PubMed]

[22] Perisic VN, Kokai G. Coeliac disease and lymphangiectasia. *Arch Dis Child.* 1992;67:134–136. [PMC free article] [PubMed]

[23] Maamer AB, Baazaoui J, Zaafouri H, Soualah W, Cherif A. Primary intestinal lymphangiectasia or Waldmann's disease: a rare cause of lower gastrointestinal bleeding. *Arab J Gastroenterol.* 2012;13:97–98. [PubMed]

[24] Macdonald J, Porter V, Scott NW, McNamara D. Small bowel lymphangiectasia and angiodysplasia: a positive association; novel clinical marker or shared pathophysiology? *J Clin Gastroenterol.* 2010;44:610–614. [PubMed]

[25] Rao R, Shashidhar H. Intestinal lymphangiectasia presenting as abdominal mass. *Gastrointest Endosc.* 2007;65:522–523, *discussion* 523. [PubMed]

[26] Kalman S, Bakkaloğlu S, Dalgiç B, Ozkaya O, Söylemezoğlu O, Buyan N. Recurrent hemolytic uremic syndrome associated with intestinal lymphangiectasia. *J Nephrol.* 2007;20:246–249. [PubMed]

[27] Dierselhuis MP, Boelens JJ, Versteegh FG, Weemaes C, Wulffraat NM. Recurrent and opportunistic infections in children with primary intestinal lymphangiectasia. *J Pediatr Gastroenterol Nutr.* 2007;44:382–385. [PubMed]

[28] Cole SL, Ledford DK, Lockey RF, Dass A, Kooper J. Primary gastrointestinal lymphangiectasia presenting as cryptococcal meningitis. *Ann Allergy Asthma Immunol.* 2007;98:490–492. [PubMed]

[29] Oehler RL, Maldonado A, Mastorides SM, Reed JL. Cryptococcalosteomyelitis complicating intestinal lymphangiectasia. *Infect Dis ClinPract.* 2007;15:125–128.

[30] Jabeen SA, Murthy A, Kandadai RM, Meena AK, Borgohain R, Uppin MS. Cryptoccocal menigitis as a primary manifestation in a patient with intestinal lymphangictasia. *Ann Indian Acad Neurol.* 2012;15:218–220. [PMC free article] [PubMed]

[31] Bouhnik Y, Etienney I, Nemeth J, Thevenot T, Lavergne-Slove A, Matuchansky C. Very late onset small intestinal B cell lymphoma associated with primary intestinal lymphangiectasia and diffuse cutaneous warts. *Gut.* 2000;47:296–300. [PMC free article] [PubMed]

[32] Bereket A, Lowenheim M, Blethen SL, Kane P, Wilson TA. Intestinal lymphangiectasia in a patient with autoimmune polyglandular disease type I and steatorrhea. *J Clin Endocrinol Metab.* 1995;80:933–935. [PubMed]

[33] Makharia GK, Tandon N, Stephen Nde J, Gupta SD, Tandon RK. Primary intestinal lymphangiectasia as a component of autoimmune polyglandular syndrome type I: a report of 2 cases. *Indian J Gastroenterol.* 2007;26:293–295. [PubMed]

[34] Alreheili K, AlMehaidib A, Alsaleem K, Banemi M, Aldekhail W, Al-Mayouf SM. Intestinal lymphangiectasia in a patient with infantile systemic hyalinosis syndrome: a rare cause of protein-losing enteropathy. *Ann Saudi Med.* 2012;32:206–208. [PubMed]

[35] Oh TG, Chung JW, Kim HM, Han SJ, Lee JS, Park JY, Song SY. Primary intestinal lymphangiectasia diagnosed by capsule endoscopy and double balloon enteroscopy. *World J Gastrointest Endosc.* 2011;3:235–240. [PMC free article] [PubMed]

[36] Gay G, Delvaux M, Frederic M. Capsule endoscopy in non-steroidal anti-inflammatory drugs-enteropathy and miscellaneous, rare intestinal diseases. *World J Gastroenterol.* 2008;14:5237–5244. [PMC free article] [PubMed]

[37] Chamouard P, Nehme-Schuster H, Simler JM, Finck G, Baumann R, Pasquali JL. Videocapsule endoscopy is useful for the diagnosis of intestinal lymphangiectasia. *Dig Liver Dis.* 2006;38:699–703. [PubMed]

[38] Asakura H, Miura S, Morishita T, Aiso S, Tanaka T, Kitahora T, Tsuchiya M, Enomoto Y, Watanabe Y. Endoscopic and histopathological study on primary and secondary intestinal lymphangiectasia. *Dig Dis Sci.* 1981;26:312–320. [PubMed]

[39] Chiu NT, Lee BF, Hwang SJ, Chang JM, Liu GC, Yu HS. Protein-losingenteropathy: diagnosis with 99mTc-labeled humanserum albumin scintigraphy. *Radiology.* 2001;219:86–90. [PubMed]

[40] So Y, Chung JK, Seo JK, Ko JS, Kim JY, Lee DS, Lee MC. Different patterns of lymphoscintigraphic findings in patients with intestinal lymphangiectasia. *Nucl Med Commun.* 2001;22:1249–1254. [PubMed]

[41] Burnand KG, McGuinness CL, Lagattolla NR, Browse NL, El-Aradi A, Nunan T. Value of isotope lymphography in the diagnosis of lymphoedema of the leg. *Br J Surg.* 2002;89:74–78. [PubMed]

[42] Steines JC, Larson JH, Wilkinson N, Kirby P, Goodheart MJ. Intestinal lymphangiectasia mimicking primary peritoneal carcinoma. *Am J Obstet Gynecol.* 2010;203:e9–e11. [PubMed]

[43] Yang DM, Jung DH. Localized intestinal lymphangiectasia: CT findings. *AJR Am J Roentgenol.* 2003;180:213–214. [PubMed]

[44] Holzknecht N, Helmberger T, Beuers U, Rust C, Wiebecke B, Reiser M. Cross-sectional imaging findings in congenital intestinal lymphangiectasia. *J Comput Assist Tomogr.* 2002;26:526–528. [PubMed]

[45] Strober W, Wochner RD, Carbone PP, Waldmann TA. Intestinal lymphangiectasia: a protein-losing enteropathy with hypogammaglobulinemia, lymphocytopenia and impaired homograft rejection. *J Clin Invest.* 1967;46:1643–1656. [PMC free article] [PubMed]

[46] Heresbach D, Raoul JL, Genetet N, Noret P, Siproudhis L, Ramée MP, Bretagne JF, Gosselin M. Immunological study in primary intestinal lymphangiectasia. *Digestion.* 1994;55:59–64. [PubMed]

[47] Fuss IJ, Strober W, Cuccherini BA, Pearlstein GR, Bossuyt X, Brown M, Fleisher TA, Horgan K. Intestinal lymphangiectasia, a disease characterized by selective loss of naive CD45RA+ lymphocytes into the gastrointestinal tract. *Eur J Immunol.* 1998;28:4275–4285. [PubMed]

[48] Vignes S, Carcelain G. Increased surface receptor Fas (CD95) levels on CD4+ lymphocytes in patients with primary intestinal lymphangiectasia. *Scand J Gastroenterol.* 2009;44:252–256. [PubMed]

[49] Davidson JD, Waldmann TA, Goodman DS, Gordon RS. Protein-losing gastroenteropathy in congestive heart-failure. *Lancet.* 1961;1:899–902. [PubMed]

[50] Valberg LS, Corbett WE, McCorriston JR, Parker JO. Excessive loss of plasma protein into the gastrointestinal tract associated with primary myocardial disease. *Am J Med.* 1965;39:668–673. [PubMed]

[51] Müller C, Globits S, Glogar D, Klepetko W, Knoflach P. Constrictive pericarditis without typical haemodynamic changes as a cause of oedema formation due to protein-losing enteropathy. *Eur Heart J.* 1991;12:1140–1143. [PubMed]

[52] Wilkinson P, Pinto B, Senior JR. Reversible protein-losing enteropathy with intestinal lymphangiectasia secondary to chronic constrictive pericarditis. *N Engl J Med.* 1965;273:1178–1181. [PubMed]

[53] Feldt RH, Driscoll DJ, Offord KP, Cha RH, Perrault J, Schaff HV, Puga FJ, Danielson GK. Protein-losing enteropathy after the Fontan operation. *J Thorac Cardiovasc Surg.* 1996;112:672–680. [PubMed]

[54] Laster L, Waldmann TA, Fenster LF, Singleton JW. Albumin metabolism in patients with Whipple's disease. *J Clin Invest.* 1966;45:637–644. [PMC free article] [PubMed]

[55] Steinfeld JL, Davidson JD, Gordon RS, Greene FE. The mechanism of hypoproteinemia in patients with regional enteritis and ulcerative colitis. *Am J Med.* 1960;29:405–415. [PubMed]

[56] Popović OS, Brkić S, Bojić P, Kenić V, Jojić N, Djurić V, Djordjević N. Sarcoidosis and protein losing enteropathy. *Gastroenterology.* 1980;78:119–125. [PubMed]

[57] Stockmann M, Fromm M, Schmitz H, Schmidt W, Riecken EO, Schulzke JD. Duodenal biopsies of HIV-infected patients with diarrhoea exhibit epithelial barrier defects but no active secretion. *AIDS.* 1998;12:43–51. [PubMed]

[58] Ploddi A, Atisook K, Hargrove NS. Intestinal lymphangiectasia in intraabdominal tuberculosis. *J Med Assoc Thai.* 1988;71:518–523. [PubMed]

[59] Rao SS, Dundas S, Holdsworth CD. Intestinal lymphangiectasia secondary to radiotherapy and chemotherapy. *Dig Dis Sci.* 1987;32:939–942. [PubMed]

[60] de Koning TJ, Dorland L, van Berge Henegouwen GP. Phosphomannoseisomerase deficiency as a cause of congenital hepatic fibrosis and protein-losing enteropathy. *J Hepatol.* 1999;31:557. [PubMed]

[61] Aoyagi K, Iida M, Matsumoto T, Sakisaka S. Enteral nutrition as a primary therapy for intestinal lymphangiectasia: value of elemental diet and polymeric diet compared with total parenteral nutrition. *Dig Dis Sci.* 2005;50:1467–1470. [PubMed]

Chapter 3

Microscopic Colitis

Abstract

Microscopic colitis (MC) is characterized by chronic, watery, secretory diarrhea, with a normal or near normal gross appearance of the colonic mucosa. Biopsy is diagnostic and usually reveals either lymphocytic colitis or collagenous colitis. The symptoms of collagenous colitis appear most commonly in the sixth decade. Patients report watery, nonbloody diarrhea of a chronic, intermittent or chronic recurrent course. With collagenous colitis, the major microscopic characteristic is a thickened collagen layer beneath the colonic mucosa, and with lymphocytic colitis, an increased number of intraepithelial lymphocytes. Histological workup can confirm a diagnosis of MC and distinguish the two distinct histological forms, namely, collagenous and lymphocytic colitis. Presently, both forms are diagnosed and treated in the same way; thus, the description of the two forms is not of clinical value although this may change in the future. Since microscopic colitis was first described in 1976 and only recently recognized as a common cause of diarrhea, many practicing physicians may not be aware of this entity. In this review, we outline the epidemiology, risk factors associated with MC, its etiopathogenesis, the approach to diagnosis and the management of these individuals.

Introduction

Microscopic colitis is regarded as one of the common causes of chronic watery diarrhea. The incidence rate for collagenous colitis is 0.8/100000-

6.2/100000. Many cases have been reported in western countries and in Asian countries like India. Lindstrom and Freeman described the term collagenous colitis concurrently in 1976. Microscopic colitis (MC) refers to two medical conditions which cause diarrhea: collagenous colitis and lymphocytic colitis. The following triad of clinicopathological features characterizes both conditions: (1) chronic watery nonbloody diarrhea; (2) normal mucosal appearance on colonoscopy; and (3) characteristic histopathology.

Patients are characteristically, although not exclusively, middle-aged females. They present with a long history of watery nonbloody diarrhea which may be profuse. There is a strong association between autoimmune diseases, for example arthritis, Sjorgen's syndrome and celiac disease, and microscopic colitis. There are reports of associations with multiple drugs, especially non-steroidal anti-inflammatory drugs. Colonoscopy is normal or near normal. The changes are often patchy, so multiple colonic biopsies must be taken in order to make a correct histological diagnosis [1-3]. A full colonoscopy is required as an examination limited to the rectum will miss cases of MC.

Epidemiology

The true incidence of MC is not known. The disease has been increasingly diagnosed over the past 20 years but is still uncommon. A recently published population-based study found the incidence of microscopic colitis to increase significantly from 1.1 per 100000 persons in the late 1980s to 19.6 per 100000 persons by the end of 2001. More recent epidemiological studies done in this century confirmed these high incidence numbers, showing that actual incidence and prevalence numbers are higher than initially thought and are still able to show rising incidences, although the rise is far less pronounced than before. Most recent north American studies show incidence rates of 7.1 per 100000 person-years for collagenous colitis and 12.6 per 100000 person-years for lymphocytic colitis [4].

Morbidity is limited to the consequences of diarrhea, including metabolic abnormalities such as hypokalemia and dehydration, weight loss and fatigue. This is not considered a life-threatening condition; however, profuse watery diarrhea may lead to severe dehydration and electrolyte abnormalities requiring intensive resuscitation.

Lymphocytic colitis affects similar numbers of men and women, while collagenous colitis is up to 20 times more frequent in women than in men [5].

Both conditions are observed most commonly in people over the age of 40 years, with peak incidence in the sixth and seventh decades of life, and the incidence of both conditions increases with age. Isolated cases have been reported in younger populations, including children [5-8].

Etiopathogenesis

The etiology of MC is most likely multifactorial with a mucosal inflammatory response to yet not specified noxious luminal agent occurring in a predisposed host. The noxious luminal agent may be a single one or multiple ones summing up to an individual threshold. Technically, MC is an inflammatory bowel disease (IBD) and the disease shares a number of etiological aspects with the so-called classical inflammatory bowel diseases like Crohn's disease and ulcerative colitis. Among the possible predisposing and/or contributing factors for microscopic colitis, genetic factors and intraluminal noxious factors are best studied. Although a limited number of familial clusters of microscopic colitis have been reported, there is only minimal evidence of a genetic component within the etiology of MC. All reported so-called family clusters are very small and comprise of a maximum of two reported family members. In contrast, there is evidence of a predisposition of sensitivity to gastrointestinal inflammatory insults in patients with microscopic colitis since up to 12% of patients with MC have a family history of celiac disease or even inflammatory bowel disease [8]. The meaning of the association between Human Leukocyte antigen (HLA-DQ2, DQ1, DQ3) and microscopic colitis and the high prevalence of a tumor necrosis factor (*TNFα*) gene polymorphisms in patients with microscopic colitis deserves further attention as it may lead to a discovery of a hereditary component of microscopic colitis of presently unknown penetration [9]. Furthermore, metalloproteinase-9 gene variations have been reported to be associated with collagenous colitis [10]. However, the meaning of all the presently reported genetic associations is poorly understood and the respective research is presently not driven by hypotheses, rather than by incidental observations or genetic screening. Very strong evidence exists for an autoimmune basis to the development of both collagenous and lymphocytic colitis. The association of MC with autoimmune-based disorders such as celiac, thyroid disease and rheumatoid arthritis, as well as the female preponderance, supports the notion that both forms of MC have a strong association with autoimmune diseases and may well be an autoimmune disorder themselves. However, to date, no specific autoantibody has been identified as being diagnostic for or being associated with collagenous or lymphocytic colitis [11]. It is known that MC can be found together with various autoantibodies and phenotypes, like human leukocyte antigen (HLA)-DR3 phenotype, although these associations are not strong enough to be regarded as being diagnostically relevant or useful, nor do we know what these associations mean. A case series of 4 patients is described in which subjects developed classic symptoms of lymphocytic-collagenous colitis with typical mucosal histopathology during treatment with omeprazole/esomeprazole (proton pump inhibitors) [12]. Symptoms promptly stopped and mucosal biopsies returned to normal with drug withdrawal. Disease quickly recurred in 2 patients who were re-exposed to the drugs, one with biopsy documented recurrent collagenous colitis. Luminal factors of whatever kind seem to play an important role in the pathogenesis of microscopic colitis. Numerous drugs were reported to have a high or at least intermediate probability of causality in microscopic colitis [13]. Other luminal factors like infectious or even toxic agents are supported by studies that found either onset of MC following a gastrointestinal infection or improvement of symptoms with the initiation of antibiotics in the context of a proven or suspected gastrointestinal infection Yesinia species [14], *Clostridium difficile* [15] and Campylobacter species [16] were suggested in published case reports to cause MC; although, interpreting these observations in the context of current knowledge, it is most likely that these cases are of sporadic nature. In some small retrospective case series, bile acid malabsorption was found in up to 60% of patients with lymphocytic and up to 44% of patients with collagenous colitis, supporting the notion that MC may at least in some patients be caused by bile acid malabsorption. Whether bile acid malabsorption is causative or not remains questionable, as later studies were unable to confirm these observations [17]. Still, this may direct therapeutic decisions and especially in patients with a cholecystectomy, a bile acid directed treatment should be considered. Basic science is still in its infancy when it comes to studying microscopic colitis and possible causes, drivers, mechanisms or even pathophysiological models. A recent bench side study employing sigmoid tissues from patients with collagenous colitis and lymphocytic colitis was able to identify that sodium transport and epithelial barrier function are disturbed in patients with microscopic colitis [18]. Unfortunately, it remains unclear whether these reported changes are of causal nature, of transient nature, or a consequence of the underlying microscopic colitis. Even although these descriptive studies at least initiate a scientific discussion on what may be mechanisms underlying or involved in the development and the resolution of microscopic colitis, these small mechanistic studies have to be carefully taken since such studies are highly artificial in the techniques they use and therefore the results are most likely influenced not only by numerous circumstances like laboratory procedures and protocols but also by patient drug use, age and even nutritional status. Thus, such information has to be considered as hypotheses generating information that hopefully guides future prospective studies that help us to understand the mechanisms involved in the pathogenesis, maintenance and resolution of microscopic colitis and symptoms associated with the histological changes.

Using molecular techniques, it was reported that in patients with MC, increased interferon-γ, TNF-α and IL-1β levels suggest a Th1 cytokine profile being involved in the inflammatory process [18]. The differences in mucosal lymphocyte subsets seen in patients with collagenous and lymphocytic colitis [19] is not fully understood presently. This information may help us to understand the inflammatory mechanisms involved and may be useful for future therapeutic approaches. Environmental factors may play a crucial role in the etiology of MC, although other than cigarette smoking, presently no other factors are confirmed. For both collagenous and lymphocytic colitis, cigarette smoking is more prevalent compared to subjects without MC and first reports suggest that lung cancer is associated with MC [20-22]. The odds ratio (OR) for lymphocytic colitis and smoking (OR = 3.8) is higher than for collagenous colitis and smoking (OR = 2.4), although this difference was calculated on a small cohort of 120 patients with collagenous colitis, 70 patients with lymphocytic colitis, and 128 controls, and thus has to be verified in larger groups of patients [23]. Interestingly, it was additionally shown that MC occurs roughly 10 years earlier when the respective person is an active smoker, stressing the relevance of cigarette smoking to the pathophysiology of microscopic colitis. Beyond the strong results from association studies, it would be of great impact to learn whether cessation of smoking would cure MC or at least be beneficial to the patient's symptoms, and a prospective clinical trial answering this seems worthwhile. In addition to the inflammatory component in the pathophysiology of MC, there may be an additional neuronal component to pathophysiology. A recent study identified increased chromogranin A, chromogranin B and secretoneurin levels in feces of patients with collagenous colitis compared to relevant control groups. These observations may point to a neurogenic involvement in MC and, additionally, these stool markers are suggested to be helpful in discriminating MC from irritable bowel syndrome or classical inflammatory bowel disease [24].

The precise mechanism of diarrhea in these patients is not well understood. Factors that may play a role include bile salt induced injury, active chloride excretion, decrease in net sodium absorption, creation of a diffusion barrier by collagen band and increased local inflammatory mediators such as nitric oxide and prostaglandins. It remains unclear which of these results in the symptoms reported by patients. Two studies have looked at inflammatory cytokines in MC. Patients with MC seem to have a predominantly TH1 type cytokine profile with significant increases in interferon gamma, TNF-α and interleukin 15, as well as an increased inducible nitric oxide synthetase. Others have found increased levels of Transforming growth factor-β in patients with collagenous colitis [25].

Clinical Presentation

Collagenous and lymphocytic colitis present with very similar symptoms and from a clinical perspective, there is no specific symptom or clinical feature that allows discriminating one from the other. Thus, the differentiation between the two entities is made by histology only. The typical clinical presentation involves chronic (either recurrent or intermittent) relapsing watery, nonbloody diarrhea. Symptoms may have been present for several months to 2-3 years before medical attention is sought and a diagnosis is made. Less frequent complaints include abdominal cramping, fecal incontinence and weight loss, although weight loss may be seen in 40% or more of patients with collagenous colitis. Incontinence is probably more a reflection of the advanced age of those individuals who are affected and patients with this problem may do well if treated with antidiarrheal agents [26, 27]. The natural history of MC is variable. Many cases are self-limiting, with symptoms lasting a few weeks or months. Others may be symptomatic for years in a relapsing or continuous pattern. Although a small number of case reports have suggested that MC may lead to development of ulcerative colitis, a small case series of patients with MC showed that none developed ulcerative colitis or Cohn's disease after a follow-up of at least 6 years [28]. There are case reports on spontaneous and colonoscopy induced colonic perforations in patients with MC [29-30].

Diagnosis/Histopathology

The diagnosis of MC is dependent on (1) a convincing clinical history with other etiologies ruled out; (2) normal or near normal endoscopic and/or radiographic findings; and (3) endoscopic biopsies with histopathological findings consistent with MC.

The first step in the diagnostic process is a thorough history with particular attention paid to risk factors and the disease associated with MC. A complete history helps one to rule out other etiologies that may cause a similar clinical picture, such as IBD, celiac disease, diarrhea-predominant irritable bowel syndrome or infectious colitis.

Laboratory and radiographic investigations can be employed to rule out other entities on the differential diagnosis list but they are typically unremarkable.

Endoscopy with biopsy is necessary to arrive at the diagnosis. Colonoscopy generally reveals normal mucosal appearance. However, non-specific changes such as erythema, edema, abnormal vascular markings or even tears associated with perforation have been described. The hallmark of microscopic colitis is an increase in inflammatory cells (*i.e.*, lymphocytes) in colonic biopsies with an otherwise normal appearance and architecture of the colon. Inflammatory cells are increased both in the surface epithelium ("intraepithelial lymphocytes") and in the lamina propria. In lymphocytic colitis, these are the only abnormal features.

In collagenous colitis, the features of lymphocytic colitis are present, with the additional presence of a characteristic thickened sub epithelial collagen band which may be up to 30 μm thick (Figure (Figure11) [31].

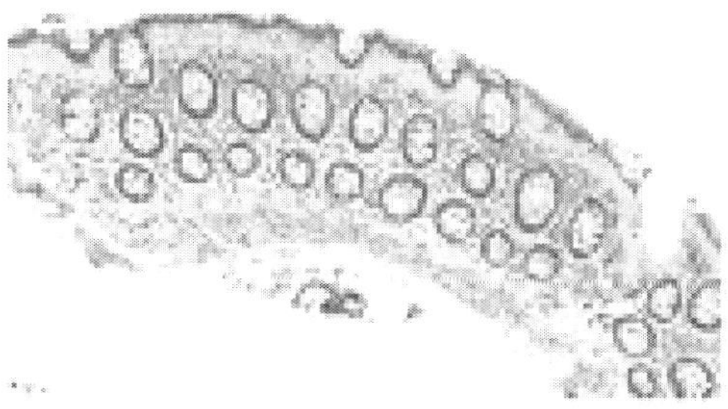

Figure 1. Micrograph of collagenous colitis, a type of microscopic colitis showing sub epithelial band of collagen H and E stain.

As the mucosa is not ulcerated or otherwise disrupted, the diarrhea generally does not contain blood or pus [32]. The diarrhea in collagenous colitis is likely due to inflammatory process and sub epithelial collagen serves as a cofactor in the role of a diffusion barrier and increased levels of immunoreactive prostaglandins E2 in stool water may lead to secretary diarrhea. Some cases may have fibrosis due to increased mucosal secretion of vascular endothelial growth factor [32, 33]. One important question is how many biopsies need to be taken and how many biopsies are needed to confirm or rule out microscopic colitis. Numerous studies showed that the microscopic lesions can be skipped and therefore random multiple colonic biopsies should be taken [34].

Treatment

Treatment recommendations for MC are largely based on case reports and uncontrolled studies. Specific agents evaluated include 5-aminosalicylic acid (5-ASA), prednisone, immunomodulators, bismuth, probiotics and *Boswellia* extract. Small randomized controlled trials have shown that agents such as budesonide offer promise as an effective form of symptomatic therapy for both collagenous and lymphocytic colitis. As a first step in managing MC, an in depth medication history should be taken with potentially precipitating medications stopped where possible. Associated conditions such as celiac disease should be appropriately managed. In patients with mild symptoms, dietary restrictions like avoiding caffeine and lactose might be helpful.

Anti-diarrheal Therapies

Non-specific anti-diarrheal therapies such as loperamide are commonly used in the management of MC. Retrospective studies have suggested benefit with doses ranging from 2 to 16 mg/d [34]. Due to the safety of this agent and the possibility of spontaneous remission, loperamide is the first-line therapy for MC.

Aminosalicylates

Uncontrolled retrospective series have suggested symptomatic improvement in up to 50% of patients with MC treated with mesalamine (5-ASA). A recent randomized trial of 64 MC patients compared mesalamine (800 mg *tid*) to mesalamine (800 mg *tid*) and cholestyramine (4 g/d). Treatment resulted in resolution of diarrhea in 84% overall after 2 wk. If treatment was continued over 6 mo, clinical and histological remission was achieved in 85% of those with lymphocytic and 91% of those with collagenous colitis. The number of relapsing patients after 6 mo of treatment was low and symptomatic relapses could be successfully retreated. Overall, the combination of mesalamine with cholestyramine was slightly superior [35, 36].

Budesonide

Budesonide is currently the most promising treatment for collagenous colitis. Three trials involving 94 patients have shown that budesonide therapy (9 mg/d for 6-8 wk) compared to placebo resulted in statistically significant improvements in clinical symptoms and quality of life. A recent Cochrane database meta-analysis reported pooled OR of 12.3 for clinical response with budesonide with a number needed to treat of two. Although effective in the short-term, all trials showed a high rate (61%-80%) of relapse within 2 wk of budesonide cessation. Age < 60 years was a significant risk factor for relapse. Although there are no studies to support a tapering course of budesonide, many clinicians employ this in an effort to minimize the likelihood of relapse.

One randomized controlled trial of budesonide for the treatment of lymphocytic colitis has been conducted. When compared to the placebo arm, the patients randomized to budesonide (9 mg/d × 6 wk) had a statistically significantly higher rate of remission (< 3 bowel movements per day) at 3 and 6 wk [37-41].

Prednisolone

A double-blind, placebo-controlled randomized trial of oral prednisolone 50 mg/d for 2 wk for collagenous colitis was inconclusive because of the low number of patients enrolled [42]. Studies examining the effect of prednisone in the treatment of lymphocytic colitis have not been performed.

Immunosuppressive Therapy

Immunosuppressive therapy with azathioprine or methotrexate has been utilized in patients either refractory to corticosteroid therapy or corticosteroid dependent, but there are no randomized controlled trials to guide therapy with these medications.

Other Therapies

Small clinical trials studying bismuth subsalicylate, *Boswellia serrata* extract, probiotics and empirical antibiotic treatment for collagenous and lymphocytic colitis look promising but cannot be suggested outside of such trials. Finally, case reports suggest that pentoxifylline, verapamil and subcutaneous octreotide might be treatment options, but their use cannot be recommended at this time. When medical therapy was unsuccessful and symptoms were very severe, surgical interventions, such as a temporary or permanent loop ileostomy or even a proctocolectomy, have been employed in smaller case series.

Conclusion

To conclude, the term microscopic colitis is now used to describe both lymphocytic and collagenous colitis and the condition should be kept in mind in any patient with unexplained watery nonbloody diarrhea with normal endoscopic findings. Biopsy is a must to rule out either form of microscopic colitis. Based on symptom severity and disease duration, a stepwise approach to treatment is suggested.

References

[1] Ingle SB, Yogesh patle, Anup kediya, Pradeep Gadgil. Collagenous colitis: cause of unexplained diarrhea. *Biomedicine*. 2012;32:279–280.

[2] Freeman HJ, Weinstein WM, SnitkaTK Watery diarrhea syndrome associated with a lesion of the colonic basement membrane (CD)-lamina propria (LP) interface. *Ann R Coll Phy Surg Can.* 1976;9:45.

[3] Fernández-Bañares F, Salas A, Esteve M, Espinós J, Forné M, Viver JM. Collagenous and lymphocytic colitis. evaluation of clinical and histological features, response to treatment, and long-term follow-up. *Am J Gastroenterol.* 2003;98:340–347. [PubMed]

[4] Pardi DS, Loftus EV, Smyrk TC, Kammer PP, Tremaine WJ, Schleck CD, Harmsen WS, Zinsmeister AR, Melton LJ, Sandborn WJ. The epidemiology of microscopic colitis: a population based study in Olmsted County, Minnesota. *Gut.* 2007;56:504–508. [PMC free article] [PubMed]

[5] Bohr J, Tysk C, Eriksson S, Abrahamsson H, Järnerot G. Collagenous colitis: a retrospective study of clinical presentation and treatment in 163 patients. *Gut.* 1996;39:846–851. [PMC free article] [PubMed]

[6] Fernández-Bañares F, Salas A, Forné M, Esteve M, Espinós J, Viver JM. Incidence of collagenous and lymphocytic colitis: a 5-year population-based study. *Am J Gastroenterol.* 1999;94:418–423. [PubMed]

[7] Olesen M, Eriksson S, Bohr J, Järnerot G, Tysk C. Microscopic colitis: a common diarrhoeal disease. An epidemiological study in Orebro, Sweden, 1993-1998. *Gut.* 2004;53:346–350. [PMC free article] [PubMed]

[8] Olesen M, Eriksson S, Bohr J, Järnerot G, Tysk C. Lymphocytic colitis: a retrospective clinical study of 199 Swedish patients. *Gut.* 2004;53:536–541. [PMC free article] [PubMed]

[9] Koskela RM, Karttunen TJ, Niemelä SE, Lehtola JK, Ilonen J, Karttunen RA. Human leucocyte antigen and TNFalpha polymorphism association in microscopic colitis. *Eur J Gastroenterol Hepatol.* 2008;20:276–282. [PubMed]

[10] Lakatos G, Sipos F, Miheller P, Hritz I, Varga MZ, Juhász M, Molnár B, Tulassay Z, Herszényi L. The behavior of matrix metalloproteinase-9 in lymphocytic colitis, collagenous colitis and ulcerative colitis. *Pathol Oncol Res.* 2012;18:85–91. [PubMed]

[11] Cindoruk M, Tuncer C, Dursun A, Yetkin I, Karakan T, Cakir N, Soykan I. Increased colonic intraepithelial lymphocytes in patients with Hashimoto's thyroiditis. *J Clin Gastroenterol.* 2002;34:237–239. [PubMed]

[12] Wilcox GM, Mattia AR. Microscopic colitis associated with omeprazole and esomeprazole exposure. *J Clin Gastroenterol.* 2009;43:551–553. [PubMed]

[13] Giardiello FM, Hansen FC, Lazenby AJ, Hellman DB, Milligan FD, Bayless TM, Yardley JH. Collagenous colitis in setting of nonsteroidal antiinflammatory drugs and antibiotics. *Dig Dis Sci.* 1990;35:257–260. [PubMed]

[14] Mäkinen M, Niemelä S, Lehtola J, Karttunen TJ. Collagenous colitis and Yersinia enterocolitica infection. *Dig Dis Sci.* 1998;43:1341–1346. [PubMed]

[15] Perk G, Ackerman Z, Cohen P, Eliakim R. Lymphocytic colitis: a clue to an infectious trigger. *Scand J Gastroenterol.* 1999;34:110–112. [PubMed]

[16] Erim T, Alazmi WM, O'Loughlin CJ, Barkin JS. Collagenous colitis associated with Clostridium difficile: a cause effect? *Dig Dis Sci.* 2003;48:1374–1375. [PubMed]

[17] Ung KA, Gillberg R, Kilander A, Abrahamsson H. Role of bile acids and bile acid binding agents in patients with collagenous colitis. *Gut.* 2000;46:170–175. [PMC free article] [PubMed]

[18] Barmeyer C, Erko I, Fromm A, Bojarski C, Allers K, Moos V, Zeitz M, Fromm M, Schulzke JD. Ion transport and barrier function are disturbed in microscopic colitis. *Ann N Y Acad Sci.* 2012;1258:143–148. [PubMed]

[19] Kumawat AK, Strid H, Elgbratt K, Tysk C, Bohr J, Hultgren Hörnquist E. Microscopic colitis patients have increased proportions of Ki67(+) proliferating and CD45RO(+) active/memory CD8(+) and CD4(+)8(+) mucosal T cells. *J Crohns Colitis.* 2013;7:694–705. [PubMed]

[20] Chan JL, Tersmette AC, Offerhaus GJ, Gruber SB, Bayless TM, Giardiello FM. Cancer risk in collagenous colitis. *Inflamm Bowel Dis.* 1999;5:40–43. [PubMed]

[21] Yen EF, Pokhrel B, Du H, Nwe S, Bianchi L, Witt B, Hall C. Current and past cigarette smoking significantly increase risk for microscopic colitis. *Inflamm Bowel Dis.* 2012;18:1835–1841. [PubMed]

[22] Bonderup OK, Folkersen BH, Gjersøe P, Teglbjaerg PS. Collagenous colitis: a long-term follow-up study. *Eur J Gastroenterol Hepatol.* 1999;11:493–495. [PubMed]

[23] Fernández-Bañares F, de Sousa MR, Salas A, Beltrán B, Piqueras M, Iglesias E, Gisbert JP, Lobo B, Puig-Diví V, García-Planella E, et al. Epidemiological risk factors in microscopic colitis: a prospective case-control study. *Inflamm Bowel Dis.* 2013;19:411–417. [PubMed]

[24] Vigren L, Sjöberg K, Benoni C, Tysk C, Bohr J, Kilander A, Larsson L, Ström M, Hjortswang H. Is smoking a risk factor for collagenous colitis? *Scand J Gastroenterol.* 2011;46:1334–1339. [PubMed]

[25] Kane J, Fischer JB. Occurrence of Trichophyton megninii in Ontario. Identification with a simple cultural procedure. *J Clin Microbiol.* 1976;2:111–114. [PMC free article] [PubMed]

[26] Freeman HJ. Long-term natural history and complications of collagenous colitis. *Can J Gastroenterol.* 2012;26:627–630. [PMC free article] [PubMed]

[27] Sylwestrowicz T, Kelly JK, Hwang WS, Shaffer EA. Collagenous colitis and microscopic colitis: the watery diarrhea-colitis syndrome. *Am J Gastroenterol.* 1989;84:763–768. [PubMed]

[28] Freeman HJ, James D, Mahoney CJ. Spontaneous peritonitis from perforation of the colon in collagenous colitis. *Can J Gastroenterol.* 2001;15:265–267. [PubMed]

[29] Bohr J, Larsson LG, Eriksson S, Järnerot G, Tysk C. Colonic perforation in collagenous colitis: an unusual complication. *Eur J Gastroenterol Hepatol.* 2005;17:121–124. [PubMed]

[30] Mullhaupt B, Güller U, Anabitarte M, Güller R, Fried M. Lymphocytic colitis: clinical presentation and long term course. *Gut.* 1998;43:629–633. [PMC free article] [PubMed]

[31] Goosenberg E. Katz J. Collagenous and Lymphocytic Colitis Treatment & Management （Medscape, 2009） Available from: http://emedicine.medscape.com/article/180664-treatment.

[32] Bamford MJ, Matz LR, Armstrong JA, Harris AR. Collagenous colitis: a case report and review of the literature. *Pathology.* 1982;14:481–484. [PubMed]

[33] Eisen GM, Dominitz JA, Faigel DO, Goldstein JA, Kalloo AN, Petersen BT, Raddawi HM, Ryan ME, Vargo JJ, Young HS, et al. Use of endoscopy in diarrheal illnesses. *Gastrointest Endosc.* 2001;54:821–823. [PubMed]

[34] Zins BJ, Tremaine WJ, Carpenter HA. Collagenous colitis: mucosal biopsies and association with fecal leukocytes. *Mayo Clin Proc.* 1995;70:430–433. [PubMed]

[35] Pardi DS, Ramnath VR, Loftus EV, Tremaine WJ, Sandborn WJ. Lymphocytic colitis: clinical features, treatment, and outcomes. *Am J Gastroenterol.* 2002;97:2829–2833. [PubMed]

[36] Calabrese C, Fabbri A, Areni A, Zahlane D, Scialpi C, Di Febo G. Mesalazine with or without cholestyramine in the treatment of

microscopic colitis: randomized controlled trial. *J Gastroenterol Hepatol.* 2007;22:809–814. [PubMed]

[37] Miehlke S, Heymer P, Bethke B, Bästlein E, Meier E, Bartram HP, Wilhelms G, Lehn N, Dorta G, DeLarive J, et al. Budesonide treatment for collagenous colitis: a randomized, double-blind, placebo-controlled, multicenter trial. *Gastroenterology.* 2002;123:978–984. [PubMed]

[38] Madisch A, Heymer P, Voss C, Wigginghaus B, Bästlein E, Bayerdörffer E, Meier E, Schimming W, Bethke B, Stolte M, et al. Oral budesonide therapy improves quality of life in patients with collagenous colitis. *Int J Colorectal Dis.* 2005;20:312–316. [PubMed]

[39] Chande N, McDonald JW, Macdonald JK. Interventions for treating lymphocytic colitis. *Cochrane Database Syst Rev.* 2008;(2):CD006096. [PubMed]

[40] Fine KD, Lee EL. Efficacy of open-label bismuth subsalicylate for the treatment of microscopic colitis. *Gastroenterology.* 1998;114:29–36. [PubMed]

[41] Munck LK, Kjeldsen J, Philipsen E, Fischer Hansen B. Incomplete remission with short-term prednisolone treatment in collagenous colitis: a randomized study. *Scand J Gastroenterol.* 2003;38:606–610. [PubMed]

[42] Pardi DS, Loftus EV, Tremaine WJ, Sandborn WJ. Treatment of refractory microscopic colitis with azathioprine and 6-mercaptopurine. *Gastroenterology.* 2001;120:1483–1484. [PubMed]

Chapter 4

Epithelial Cysts of the Spleen: A Minireview

Abstract

Primary splenic epithelial cyst is an unusual event in everyday surgical practice with about 800 cases reported until date in the English literature. Splenic cysts may be parasitic or non-parasitic in origin. Nonparasitic cysts are either primary or secondary. Primary cysts are also called true, congenital, epidermoid or epithelial cysts. Primary splenic cysts account for 10% of all benign non-parasitic splenic cysts and are the most frequent type of splenic cysts in children. Usually, splenic cysts are asymptomatic and can be found incidentally during imaging techniques or on laprotomy. The symptoms are related to the size of cysts. When they assume large sizes, they may present with fullness in the left abdomen, local or referred pain, symptoms due to compression of adjacent structures (like nausea, vomiting, flatulence, diarrhoea) or rarely thrombocytopenia, and occasionally complications such as infection, rupture and/or haemorrhage. The preoperative diagnosis of primary splenic cysts can be ascertained by ultrasonography (USG), computed tomography or magnetic resonance imaging, although the wide use of USG today has led to an increase in the incidence of splenic cysts by 1%. However, careful histopathological evaluation along with immunostaining for presence of epithelial lining is mandatory to arrive at the diagnosis. The treatment has changed drastically from total splenectomy in the past to splenic preservation methods recently.

Introduction

Primary splenic cysts are unusual and often an incidental finding in surgical practice. As per the existing literature, since the first case was reported in 1929 by Andral, the classification of these lesions has evolved into the present system [1].

Classification

Splenic cysts have been classified based on the presence or absence of an epithelial lining, etiology, pathogenesis, etc. Martin classified splenic cysts as type 1 cysts, which are true cysts having lining epithelium, and type 2 cysts, which are false cysts without lining epithelium [2, 3]. Pseudocysts are usually posttraumatic, due to failure of organization of hematomas located beneath the capsule or in the splenic parenchyma, and rarely they may occur in splenic abscess or splenic infarction [1, 4, 5]. Depending on the causative agent splenic cysts can be divided into two types: parasitic cysts and non-parasitic cysts. Parasitic cysts are usually seen in endemic areas and are caused mainly by *Echinococcus granulosus* infestation [1, 6, 7]. A new classification based on the true pathogenesis of cyst divides non-parasitic splenic cysts as congenital, neoplastic, traumatic, and degenerative [8]. Primary splenic cysts constitute 10% of all nonparasitic cysts of the spleen. These cysts are predominantly seen in paediatric and adolescent age groups [2, 9]. Usually they are asymptomatic and found incidentally on ultrasound examination of the abdomen [2]. The clinical significance is attributed mainly because of their potential to rupture, to infect or to bleed, and due to the potential of a serious differential diagnosis of a neoplastic lesion in the left hypochondrium [10].

Recently, treatment of choice is open partial splenectomy as it preserves the splenic functions and there is no recurrence of the lesion due to complete removal [11]. Histopathological evaluation along with immunohistochemistry is the mainstay to confirm the subtype of splenic cyst and to rule out the rare possibility of malignant transformation in the pluripotent epithelial lining [12].

Epidemiology

Primary splenic epithelial cyst is a rare condition with an incidence rate of 0.07% as reported in a review of 42327 autopsies [13-16]. Primary splenic cysts are seen mostly in children, adolescents and young adults [13]. Congenital type is common in girls [17, 18]. Non-parasitic splenic cysts are common in Europe and North America, while parasitic cysts are common in Africa and Central America [19]. The prevalence rate of splenic cysts has been increased nowadays due to increased use of non-invasive diagnostic modalities, i.e., ultrasonography (USG) and computed tomography (CT) [20].

Pathophysiology

The pathogenesis of primary splenic cysts is not clear. In view of this, many hypotheses were proposed.

Mesothelial invagination Theory

In case of congenital cysts, it is postulated that during development there is invasion of mesothelial lining along with the capsule. As the lining has pluripotent nature, it has propensity to undergo metaplasia and secretion of fluid, leading to the formation of cysts [1, 5].

The congenital cyst lining is postulated to arise from invasion of the peritoneum along with its mesothelial lining after rupture of the splenic capsule or due to trapping of mesothelial cells in splenic sulci.

Lymph Space Theory

According to this theory the cysts may arise from the normal lymph spaces in the spleen [16].

Endodermal Inclusion Theory

Endodermal inclusion theory proposes that epithelial splenic cysts develop by true metaplasia of a heterotopic endodermal inclusion within the spleen [21-23]. Due to pluripotent nature of the mesothelium, there seems to be metaplasia in the lining leading to formation of cysts with various types of epithelial lining, i.e., squamous, columnar, etc. [12]. According to some studies the epidermoid nature is due to teratomatous differentiation or to inclusion of fetal squamous lining instead of metaplasia.

Clinical Features

Age

Splenic cysts are predominantly seen in the second and third decades; however, they can be seen in paediatric age group [24].

Sex

Splenic cysts are common in females as compared to males [18].

Signs and Symptoms

Usually small cysts are symptomless. A painless mass in the left hypochondriac region is the main presentation in 30%-40% cases. There may be localized pain or referred pain due to mass effect [25]. Occasionally the patients may present with thrombocytopenia [1, 26]. The initial symptoms are mainly due to pressure effect, including nausea and belching pain in the abdomen [25]. Pleuritic pain and persistent cough are also the presenting features [27]. Occasionally they present with complications, like infection, rupture and haemorrhage [25, 28]. Physical examination often reveals a left hypochondriac mass. The routine haematological and biochemical investigations are within normal limits.

Tumour Markers

The serum tumour markers carcinoembryonic antigen (CEA) and carbohydrate antigen 19-9 (CA 19-9) may be raised and so checked [29].

Diagnosis

Clinical Diagnosis

Most of primary cysts are clinically silent and are diagnosed incidentally on USG. Nowadays, the prevalence is increased because of the increased use of non-invasive imaging techniques, i.e., USG and CT [30].

Whenever there is a lump in the left hypochondriac region, the clinician should exclude other causes of splenomegaly, i.e., infectious mononucleosis, fever of unknown origin, haemolytic anaemia, chronic leukaemias, collagen vascular disease, and liver diseases. Serological markers play key role in such circumstances [31].

USG

USG is a good non-invasive tool for screening and confirming the cystic nature of a mass [2]. Ultrasound can differentiate solid and cystic lesions in most cases [32]. Characteristically, on USG the cyst appears as an anechoic mass with thin walls and septations or irregular walls. There are calcific foci in case of complex cysts. Calcifications are useful to differentiate cysts from other causes of splenomegaly [27, 30, 10].

CT and Magnetic Resonance Imaging

CT and magnetic resonance imaging (MRI) may give guidelines, with regard to the morphology of cyst, the nature of fluid, the exact location and its relationship with adjacent structures [10, 27, 30]. On T1-weighted MRI images, the cyst is hypointense while on T2, it is hyperintense, with intensity of signal equal to water without reinforcement after contrast injection. However, the signal intensity may be elevated according to contents in the cyst, e.g., signal intensity on T1 can be increased in case of a hemorrhagic cyst [33].

Accurate Clinical Diagnosis

Accurate clinical diagnosis of primary epithelial cysts is difficult; the occurrence of a unilocular cyst in the absence of previous trauma, infection or exposure to hydatid disease may help to arrive at the diagnosis [1]. The diagnosis of pseudocyst should be suspected in cases with a history of trauma, elder age along with evidence of hematoma in the organ parenchyma and calcification in the cyst wall. The diagnosis of hydatid cyst is done by detailed clinical history, the evidence of calcification in the wall, and presence of daughter cysts with multiple organ involvement [34, 35].

Other Techniques

Other techniques such as 99m technetium sulphur colloid scintigraphy and 67-gallium citrate also prove the diagnostic utility [2]. The inner cyst wall is immunoreactive to anti-CA 19-9 antibodies [36]. Serum levels of the markers may be low as compared to actual elevations within the cystic cavity.

Angiography is helpful in differentiating a splenic cyst, which is usually an avascular lesion, while the malignant tumours (lymphoma, sarcoma) usually have a disarranged vascular pattern [27, 13].

However, definite diagnosis is possible only after splenectomy when epithelial lining is confirmed by histopathology along with immunohistochemistry. Primary epithelial cysts are usually solitary, but can be multiple. Cases have also been described in accessory spleens [37, 38].

The cysts are either unilocular/multilocular with occasional calcific foci. Figure 1 shows an example of a unilocular cyst with smooth glistening inner wall surface.

Histologically, primary splenic cysts have epithelial lining, i.e., flattened, low cuboidal, low columnar or squamous type and unilayered or multilayered with benign nuclear features [1]. Epidermoid cysts have stratified squamous epithelium with a fibrocollagenous cyst wall (Figure 3). Immunohistochemically, the epithelial cells are positive for pan-cytokeratin and negative for CD240 (a lymphatic epithelial marker) and CD34 (an endothelial cell marker). Figure 4 shows an example of primary splenic cyst lined with cuboidal to flattened epithelium.

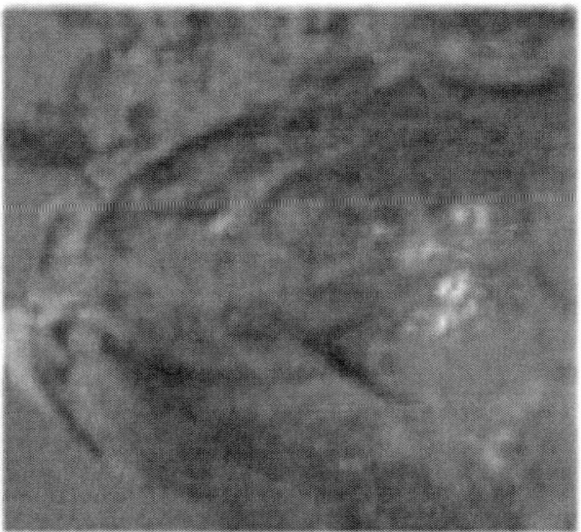

Figure 1. Huge primary splenic cyst with glistening smooth inner wall.

A case of multilocular primary epithelial cyst of the spleen in a postmenopausal women presenting as splenomegaly was reported (Figure 2) [12].

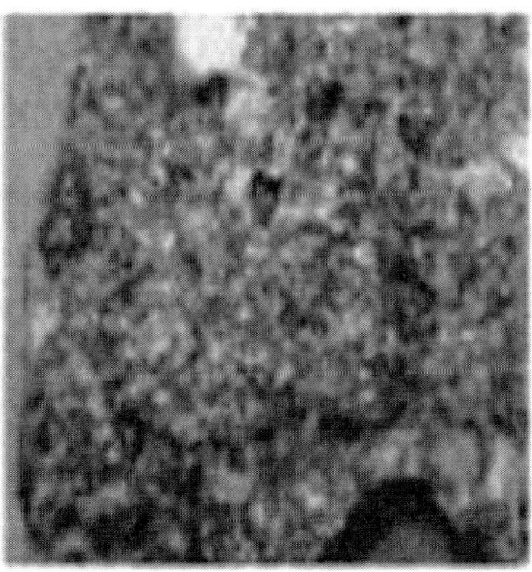

Figure 2. Multiloculated primary splenic cyst.

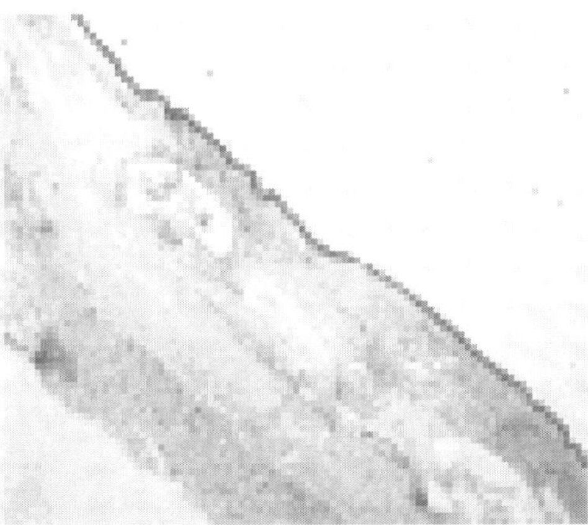

Figure 3. Epidermoid cyst of the spleen (Hematoxylin and eosin staining, × 10).

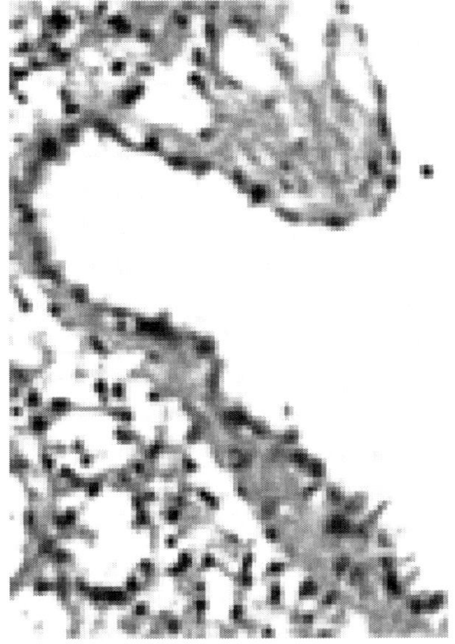

Figure 4. Primary splenic cyst lined with cuboidal to flattened epithelium (Hematoxylin and eosin staining, × 10).

The differential diagnoses for a cysts in the spleen include parasitic echinococcal disease, congenital cyst, posttraumatic pseudocyst, infarction, infection, pyogenic splenic abscess, pancreatic pseudocyst, metastatic disease, and cystic neoplasms like haemangioma/lymphangioma (diffuse lymphangiomatosis of spleen) (Figure 5).

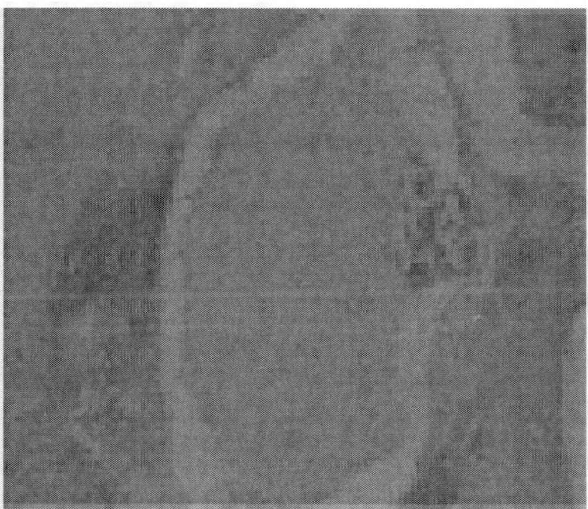

Figure 5. Diffuse lymphangiomatosis of the spleen (Hematoxylin and eosin staining, × 10).

Treatment

Previously, splenectomy was the treatment of choice for splenic cysts. Recently, the approach is changed towards conservative surgery in view of overwhelming sepsis after splenectomy leading to raised mortality. The splenic cysts with a diameter more than 4 cm should be treated surgically [11]. Traditionally the cysts have been treated either by partial or total splenectomy. However, there are chances of overwhelming sepsis after splenectomy. In the modern era of laparoscopic surgery, more interest in conservative surgery like percutaneous aspiration and sclerosis is documented to prevent post splenectomy complications. Marsupialisation is very much effective in small cysts.

There are different types of surgical modalities according to thc clinical situation.

Today, there are different conservative treatment modalities, including percutaneous drainage, partial splenectomy with a stapler or harmonic scalpel, total cystectomy, marsupialisation or cyst unroofing. Laparoscopic puncture and creation of a cyst peritoneal window are also an effective conservative treatment modality. The aim of partial splenectomy is to retain the immunological protection of patient by preserving more than 25% of the splenic parenchyma, which is the optimum splenic tissue to preserve immunologic efficiency without increasing the risk of recurrence [28].

Any type of conservative surgical treatment modality has little value in cases such as a very large cyst in the hilum of the spleen, an intrasplenic cyst almost surrounded by splenic parenchyma, with dense vascular adhesions to surrounding structures, and multiple cysts. In such circumstances, splenectomy either by open approach or by laparoscopic approach is the treatment of choice.

Prognosis

The clinical importance of splenic cysts is due to their potential to rupture, to be infected or to bleed. Cysts with a diameter > 5 cm are more likely to rupture resulting in life threatening haemoperitoneum. Two rare cases of patients with epithelial splenic cysts as an incidental finding during emergency laprotomy for splenic rupture were reported [39]. The most common infection is caused by Salmonella bacteria [13]. A 12-year-old prepubertal gir presenting with a large congenital splenic cyst complicated by *Salmonella* infection was documented [18]. Pregnancy associated splenic cysts are extremely rare and only five cases were described [40]. A case of squamous cell carcinoma in an epidermoid cyst was reported in a pregnant woman [4].

References

[1] Ingle SB, Hinge CR, Jatal SN. An interesting case of primary epithelial cyst of spleen. *Indian J Pathol Microbiol.* 2013;56:181–182. [PubMed]

[2] Garg M, Kataria SP, Sethi D, Mathur SK. Epidermoid cyst of spleen mimicking splenic lymphangioma. *Adv Biomed Res.* 2013;2:49. [PMC free article] [PubMed]

[3] Martin JW. Congenital splenic cysts. *Am J Surg.* 1958;96:302–308. [PubMed]

[4] Schwarts SI. The spleen. In: Schwartz SI, Harold E, editors. Maingot's Abdominal Operations. 9th edition. USA: Appleton and Lange; 1990. p. 80.

[5] Valente AP, Barrabin H, Jorge RV, Paes MC, Scofano HM. Isolation and characterization of the Mg2(+)-ATPase from rabbit skeletal muscle

sarcoplasmic reticulum membrane preparations. *Biochim Biophys Acta.* 1990;1039:297–304. [PubMed]

[6] Avital S, Kashtan H. A large epithelial splenic cyst. *N Engl J Med.* 2003;349:2173–2174. [PubMed]

[7] Kalinova K. Giant pseudocyst of the spleen: A case report and review of the literature. *J Indian Assoc Pediatr Surg.* 2005;10:176–178.

[8] Morgenstern L. Nonparasitic splenic cysts: pathogenesis, classification, and treatment. *J Am Coll Surg.* 2002;194:306–314. [PubMed]

[9] Belekar D, Desai A, Dewoolkar A, Dewoolkar V, Bhutala U. Splenic epithelial cyst: A rare entity. *Int J Surg.* 2010;22:1–18.

[10] Hansen MB, Moller AC. Splenic cysts. *Surg Laparosc Endosc Percutan Tech.* 2004;14:316–322. [PubMed]

[11] Szczepanik AB, Meissner AJ. Partial splenectomy in the management of nonparasitic splenic cysts. *World J Surg.* 2009;33:852–856. [PubMed]

[12] Manoj MG, Misra P, Kakkar S. Multilocular epithelial cyst of spleen: a rare occurrence. *Indian J Pathol Microbiol.* 2012;55:602–604. [PubMed]

[13] Macheras A, Misiakos EP, Liakakos T, Mpistarakis D, Fotiadis C, Karatzas G. Non-parasitic splenic cysts: a report of three cases. *World J Gastroenterol.* 2005;11:6884–6887. [PubMed]

[14] Doolas A, Nolte M, McDonald OG, Economou SG. Splenic cysts. *J Surg Oncol.* 1978;10:369–387. [PubMed]

[15] Geraghty M, Khan IZ, Conlon KC. [In Process Citation] *J Minim Access Surg.* 2009;5:14–16. [PMC free article] [PubMed]

[16] Robbins FG, Yellin AE, Lingua RW, Craig JR, Turrill FL, Mikkelsen WP. Splenic epidermoid cysts. *Ann Surg.* 1978;187:231–235. [PMC free article] [PubMed]

[17] Hilmes MA, Strouse PJ. The pediatric spleen. *Semin Ultrasound CT MR.* 2007;28:3–11. [PubMed]

[18] Karia N, Lakhoo K. Complicated congenital splenic cyst: saved by a splenunculus. *Afr J Paediatr Surg.* 2011;8:98–100. [PubMed]

[19] Sellers GJ, Starker PM. Laparoscopic treatment of a benign splenic cyst. *Surg Endosc.* 1997;11:766–768. [PubMed]

[20] Wu HM, Kortbeek JB. Management of splenic pseudocysts following trauma: a retrospective case series. *Am J Surg.* 2006;191:631–634. [PubMed]

[21] Kundal VK, Gajdhar M, Kundal R, Sharma C, Agrawal D, Meena A. Giant Epithelial Non-Parasitic Splenic *Cyst. J Case Rep.* 2013;3:106–109.

[22] Harding HE. A large inclusion cyst in a spleen. *J Path.* 1933;36:485.

[23] Touloukian RJ, Maharaj A, Ghoussoub R, Reyes M. Partial decapsulation of splenic epithelial cysts: studies on etiology and outcome. *J Pediatr Surg.* 1997;32:272–274. [PubMed]

[24] Sakamoto Y, Yunotani S, Edakuni G, Mori M, Iyama A, Miyazaki K. Laparoscopic splenectomy for a giant splenic epidermoid cyst: report of a case. *Surg Today.* 1999;29:1268–1272. [PubMed]

[25] Trompetas V, Panagopoulos E, Priovolou-Papaevangelou M, Ramantanis G. Giant benign true cyst of the spleen with high serum level of CA 19-9. *Eur J Gastroenterol Hepatol.* 2002;14:85–88. [PubMed]

[26] Tsakraklides V, Hadley TW. Epidermoid cysts of the spleen. A report of five cases. *Arch Pathol.* 1973;96:251–254. [PubMed]

[27] Labruzzo C, Haritopoulos KN, El Tayar AR, Hakim NS. Posttraumatic cyst of the spleen: a case report and review of the literature. *Int Surg.* 2002;87:152–156. [PubMed]

[28] Till H, Schaarschmidt K. Partial laparoscopic decapsulation of congenital splenic cysts. A medium-term evaluation proves the efficiency in children. *Surg Endosc.* 2004;18:626–628. [PubMed]

[29] Walz MK, Metz KA, Sastry M, Eigler FW, Leder LD. Benign mesothelial splenic cyst may cause high serum concentration of CA 19-9. *Eur J Surg.* 1994;160:389–391. [PubMed]

[30] Robertson F, Leander P, Ekberg O. Radiology of the spleen. *Eur Radiol.* 2001;11:80–95. [PubMed]

[31] Knudson P, Coon W, Schnitzer B, Liepman M. Splenomegaly without an apparent cause. *Surg Gynecol Obstet.* 1982;155:705–708. [PubMed]

[32] Siniluoto TM, Päivänsalo MJ, Lähde ST, Alavaikko MJ, Lohela PK, Typpö AB, Suramo IJ. Nonparasitic splenic cysts. Ultrasonographic features and follow-up. *Acta Radiol.* 1994;35:447–451. [PubMed]

[33] Ramani M, Reinhold C, Semelka RC, Siegelman ES, Liang L, Ascher SM, Brown JJ, Eisen RN, Bret PM. Splenic hemangiomas and hamartomas: MR imaging characteristics of 28 lesions. *Radiology.* 1997;202:166–172. [PubMed]

[34] Fernández-Ruiz M, Guerra-Vales JM, Enguita-Valls AB, Vila-Santos J, García-Borda FJ, Morales-Gutiérrez C. Splenic hydatid cyst, a rare location of extrahepatic echinococcosis: Report of six cases. *Eur J Intern Med.* 2008;19:e51–e53. [PubMed]

[35] Polat P, Kantarci M, Alper F, Suma S, Koruyucu MB, Okur A. Hydatid disease from head to toe. *Radiographics.* 2003;23:475–494; quiz 536-537. [PubMed]

[36] Madia C, Lumachi F, Veroux M, Fiamingo P, Gringeri E, Brolese A, Zanus G, Cillo U, D'Amico DF. Giant splenic epithelial cyst with elevated serum markers CEA and CA 19-9 levels: an incidental association? *Anticancer Res.* 2003;23:773–776. [PubMed]

[37] Morohoshi T, Hamamoto T, Kunimura T, Yoshida E, Kanda M, Funo K, Nagayama T, Maeda M, Araki S. Epidermoid cyst derived from an accessory spleen in the pancreas. A case report with literature survey. *Acta Pathol Jpn.* 1991;41:916–921. [PubMed]

[38] Tateyama H, Tada T, Murase T, Fujitake S, Eimoto T. Lymphoepithelial cyst and epidermoid cyst of the accessory spleen in the pancreas. *Mod Pathol.* 1998;11:1171–1177. [PubMed]

[39] Fragandreas G, Papadopoulos S, Gerogiannis I, Spyridis C, Tsantilas D, Venizelos I, Gerasimidis T. Epithelial splenic cysts and life-threatening splenic rupture. *Chirurgia* (Bucur) 2011;106:519–522. [PubMed]

[40] Rotas M, Ossowski R, Lutchman G, Levgur M. Pregnancy complicated with a giant splenic cyst: a case report and review of the literature. *Arch Gynecol Obstet.* 2007;275:301–305. [PubMed]

Chapter 5

Crohn's Disease of Stomach and Duodenum

Abstract

Crohn's disease (CD) is a chronic idiopathic inflammatory disease of gastrointestinal tract characterized by segmental and transmural involvement of gastrointestinal tract. Ileocolonic and colonic/anorectal is a most common and account for 40% of cases and involvement of small intestine is about 30%. Isolated involvement of stomach is an extremely unusual presentation of the disease accounting for less than 0.07% of all gastrointestinal CD. To date there are only a few documented case reports of adults with isolated gastric CD and no reports in the pediatric population. The diagnosis is difficult to establish in such cases with atypical presentation. In the absence of any other source of disease and in the presence of nonspecific upper GI endoscopy and histological findings, serological testing can play a vital role in the diagnosis of atypical CD. Recent studies have suggested that perinuclear anti-neutrophil cytoplasmic antibody *(PNCA)* and anti-*Saccharomycescervisia* antibody *(ASCA)* may be used as additional diagnostic tools. The effectiveness of infliximab in isolated gastric CD is limited to only a few case reports of adult patients and the long-term outcome is unknown.

Introduction

CD is a chronic inflammatory disease of the gastrointestinal tract that can involve any part of the gastrointestinal tract from mouth to the anus. In majority of the patients, multiple lesions are seen but isolated gastric CD is an extremely unusual event in clinical practice. In common presentations, the diagnosis of CD is easy and usually based on a combination of typical clinical, laboratory, endoscopic and pathological findings. The ASCA is a marker for CD with relatively good specificity but poor sensitivity. However, the diagnosis is difficult to establish in cases with atypical presentation as in an isolated gastroduodenal disease. In such a scenario other possible etiologies must be systematically ruled out in order to establish the correct pathological diagnosis [1, 2].

The most well known criteria for the diagnosis of gastroduodenal Crohn's disease are those of *Nugent and Roy,* which include either

1. Histological finding of noncaseating granulomatous inflammation of the stomach or duodenum, with or without concomitant CD in the remaining gastrointestinal tract, *and* the absence of other systemic granulomatous disorders; or
2. Confirmed Crohn's disease of the gastrointestinal tract *and* radiographic or endoscopic findings of diffuse inflammation of the stomach or duodenum consistent with CD [3-9].

Epidemiology

Incidence-Clinically significant gastroduodenal CD occurs in 0.5% to 4% of all patients with CD [3-6]. Isolated stomach involvement is very unusual presentation accounting for less than 0.07% of all gastrointestinal CD [1].

Pattern of involvement- Most patients have associated involvement of distal small or large intestine [7]. One third of patients with gastroduodenal Crohn's disease do not have small or large bowel disease at the time of diagnosis but develop distal disease over a period of time [8]. Prospective studies of patients with intestinal Crohn's disease have identified upper gastrointestinal abnormalities through double-contrast radiography in 20% to 40%, through endoscopy in 20% to 30%, and through histology in 30% to 50% of patients [4, 9]. Contiguous gastroduodenal involvement is the most common pattern, with about 60% of patients having diseased antrum, pylorus, and proximal duodenum [6, 10, 11].

Age-The mean age of presentation is the third and fourth decades [6]. The age of presentation varies, and cases are reported in both adults and children.

Sex predilection- Gastroduodenal Crohn's disease is noted almost equally in men and women, with a 1.2:1 ratio [6, 12].

Pathophysiology

For pathogenesis of isolated gastric CD multiple hypothesis were postulated

1. The *"hygiene hypothesis"* has been proposed as the probable underlying reason for the switch from infectious to chronic inflammatory diseases and it postulates that there has been a fundamental lifestyle change from one with high microbial exposure to one with low microbial exposure [13]. A relative lack of microbial antigens early in life would lead to a less educated and weaker immune system, not equipped to properly handle new challenges later on in life and generating an ineffective immune response that is prolonged because it is powerless to eliminate the offending agent.

A variety of *environmental factors* are considered risk factors for IBD, including smoking, diet, drugs, geography and social status, stress, the enteric flora, altered intestinal permeability and appendectomy [14]. Among them, cigarette smoking is the strongest example of the influence of the environment on IBD.

Immune mechanism- In CD, intestinal CD4+ T cells produce large amounts of most IBD patients show an enhanced systemic and mucosal immunological reactivity against gut bacterial antigens. Among these, based on serum antibody titers, *bacterial flagellin* has been recently reported as a dominant antigen in CD [15], apparently defining a population of patients with complicated CD [16]. It has been proposed that this immune reactivity is the consequence of a *'loss of tolerance'* towards the autologous enteric flora, resulting in an inappropriate immune response in the mucosa which is manifested by the chronic inflammatory process typical of Crohn's disease.

Role of chemical mediators-INF-γ and marked overexpression of the Th1-cell-specific transcription factor, T-bet [17], while mucosal macrophages produce large amounts of IL-12 and IL-18 [18, 19]. Additionally, CD mucosal T-cells are resistant to apoptosis and cycle faster than control cells [20, 21]. Based on these observations, it is now generally accepted CD is associated with distinct immune profiles which is classified as a fairly typical Th1 response in CD. Different types of immunoregulatory cells exist, the best defined being CD4 + CD25 high T-cells, which are critically important in preventing autoimmunity and suppressing excessive immune reactivity [22]. In CD there is a contraction of this regulatory cell pool in the blood and only a moderate expansion in the inflamed intestine, suggesting the presence of insufficient regulation during active disease [23].

Role of mucosal dendritic cells -In IBD, mucosal dendritic cells are activated, express increased levels of the toll-like receptors (TLR) 2 and TLR4- which mediate recognition of bacterial products - and CD40, and produce more IL-12 and IL-6 [24]. All of these phenotypic and functional features indicate a prominent role of dendritic cells in IBD pathogenesis.

Epithelial cells- are also involved in innate immunity. Interestingly, ileal Paneth cells also express the NOD2 protein, and their production of mucosal α-defensins is decreased in CD patients with NOD2 mutations, perhaps leading to an impaired resistance against enteric microorganisms and eventually contributing to bacteria-induced inflammation [25].

To conclude, we appear to have settled down on a unifying but still wide-ranging hypothesis that IBD results from complex interactions between evolving environmental changes induced by society's progress, a still undefined number of predisposing genetic mutations, an incredibly complex gut microbiota that may be constantly varying, and the intricacies of individual immune systems [26].

Clinical Presentations

1. *Age*-The mean age of presentation is the third and fourth decades [6]. The age of presentation varies, and cases are reported in both adults and children.

Sex predilection- Gastroduodenal Crohn's disease is noted almost equally in men and women, with a 1.2:1 ratio [6, 12].

Symptoms and signs- Most patients with gastroduodenal Crohn's disease are asymptomatic from the gastroduodenal involvement [9]. The most common symptom is epigastric abdominal pain, which is often postprandial in timing, nonradiating, and usually relieved by food and antacids [4, 9, 11]. Pronounced, continuous abdominal pain associated with nausea and vomiting suggests gastric outlet obstruction due to gastroduodenal stricture formation [4]. Other common symptoms include profound weight loss, nausea with or without vomiting, and anorexia [4, 9, 27]. Symptoms may be wrongly attributed to peptic ulcer disease or a side effect of drug therapy (i.e., 5-aminosalicylic acid, prednisone, 6-mercaptopurine, azathioprine, or metronidazole) [4]. Gastrointestinal blood loss may be noted in gastroduodenal Crohn's disease, usually in the form of chronic anemia, although melena and hematemesis indicating acute hemorrhage may rarely occur [4, 9, 11, 27].

Uncommon presentations of CD may manifest as a single symptom or sign, such as impairment of linear growth, delayed puberty, perianal disease, mouth ulcers, clubbing, chronic iron deficiency anemia or extra-intestinal manifestations preceding the gastrointestinal symptoms, mainly arthritis or arthralgia, primary sclerosing cholangitis, pyoderma gangrenosum and rarely osteoporosis [2]. In such cases, the diagnosis is challenging and can remain elusive for some time.

Diagnostic Evaluation

In common presentations, the diagnosis of Crohn's disease is usually based on a combination of typical clinical, laboratory, endoscopic and pathological findings. However, the diagnosis is difficult to establish in cases of atypical presentation as in isolated gastroduodenal disease. In such a scenario other possible etiologies must be systematically ruled out in order to establish the diagnosis. These may include *Helicobacter pylori* infection, tuberculosis, non-steroidal anti-inflammatory drugs, eosinophilic gastritis, Menetrier's disease, gastrinoma, collagen vascular disease, and lymphoma. Additional diagnostic strategy in atypical cases of inflammatory bowel disease is the use of anti-*Saccharomyces cervisia* antibody (*ASCA)*. This serological marker can be a helpful adjunctive tool in the diagnostic process despite the test's limitations [2].

2. *Radiological signs* - The earliest radiographic sign in Crohn's disease are aphthous ulcers [28]. The most common radiologic findings in gastroduodenal Crohn's disease are mucosal nodularity, or "cobblestoning," thickened folds, and ulcerations [4]. A pseudo-Billroth I appearance of involved antrum and proximal duodenum can also be seen [4, 12]. A rare but classic radiographic finding is the funnel-shaped deformity of diseased antrum and duodenal bulb, known as the *"ram's horn"* sign [7, 28]. Radiographic evaluation with double-contrast medium is the best modality to assess lesions

that have formed stenoses or strictures, which are findings of advanced disease [6, 12, 27, 29, 30]. A barium enema should be done when a gastrocolic fistula is suspected, as this has a higher sensitivity than upper gastrointestinal radiography [4].

3. Endoscopy - Endoscopy with biopsy, is an effective tool for surveying the mucosa & remains the gold standard in the diagnosis of gastroduodenal Crohn's disease and is most likely to identify early gastric and/or duodenal involvement [6, 9, 27, 30]. Endoscopic findings include patchy erythema, gastric outlet narrowing (Figure 1) mucosal friability, thickened folds, and ulcerations, both aphthous and linear [4, 7, 9, 12]. Unlike peptic ulcers, those of gastroduodenal Crohn's disease are not usually circular but linear or serpiginous [27]. Another common endoscopic feature, characteristic but not specific, is a nodular mucosa (cobble stoning) [7, 9, 12]. A linitis plastica appearance, with luminal narrowing and rigidity, and thickened folds suggest diffuse gastric involvement [31, 32].

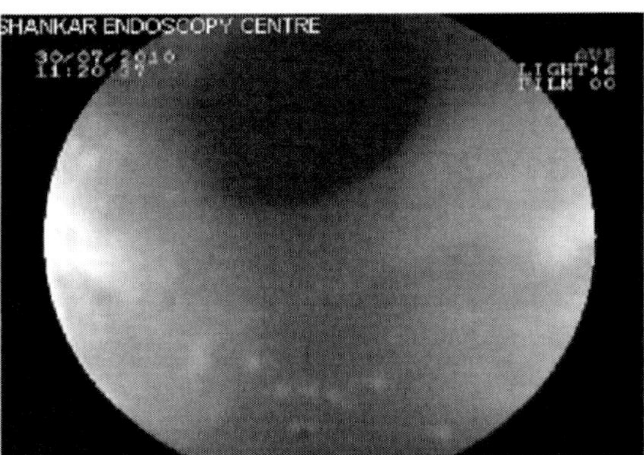

Figure 1. Endoscopic findings include patchy erythema, gastric outlet narrowing.

4. *Biopsy findings* - The histologic findings of gastroduodenal Crohn's disease are often nonspecific and have a patchy distribution. To exclude other diagnoses, multiple biopsies should be taken from the stomach and duodenum. Noncaseating granulomas *are* seen in 5% to 83% of gastroduodenal biopsies in Crohn's disease (figures 2 and 3) and therefore may not be present [9, 12]. Granulomas can be seen in a number of other diseases, including *H. pylori* infection, peptic ulcer disease complications, gastric carcinoma, gastric lymphoma, sarcoidosis, tuberculosis, syphilis, hypertrophic gastropathy,

eosinophilic gastritis, Wegener's granulomatosis, food and suture granulomas , histoplasmosis, Whipple's disease, and the controversial diagnosis of idiopathic isolated granulomatous gastritis, to name only a few [7, 9, 32]. Therefore, the finding of granulomatous gastritis is not specific for Crohn's disease.

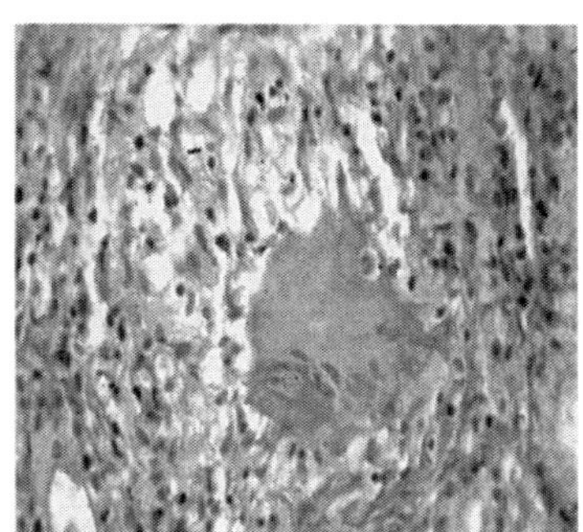

Figure 2.

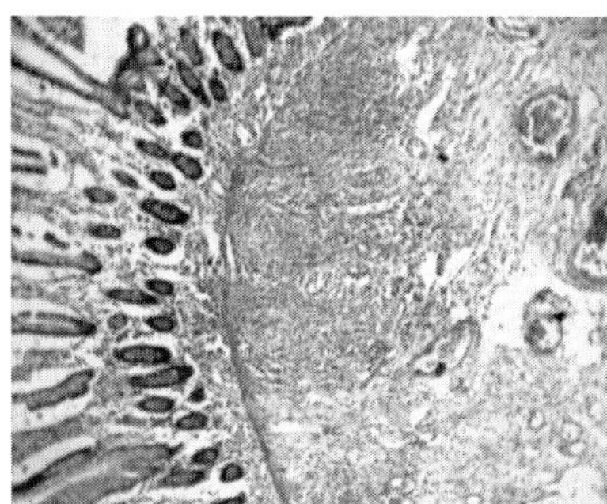

Figure 3.

Figures 2 and 3. Photomicrograph of Crohn's Disease showing non-caseating granulomas and oedema in the submucosa (H & E; 10x X 10x).

The most common pathologic finding encountered in gastric Crohn's disease is *H. pylori*–negative focal patchy gastritis, or focally enhanced gastritis, with or without granulomas, noted in 76% of patients with known Crohn's disease of the small and/ or large intestine [7, 9, 33-35]. Characterized by focal infiltration of lymphocytes and histiocytes, this focally enhanced gastritis has no correlation with clinical and laboratory findings [32]. It should be noted that the prevalence of *H. pylori* in patients with Crohn's disease is similar to that in the general population [4]. Additional histologic features include mucosal edema, acute or chronic inflammation, crypt abscesses, lymphoid aggregates, erosions, ulcers, abnormal villi, and fibrosis extending into the muscularis mucosa [32, 33].

5. *Serological markers* - Recent studies have suggested that perinuclear anti-neutrophil cytoplasmic antibody *(pANCA)* and *ASCA* may be used as additional diagnostic tools for patients with suspected inflammatory bowel disease and help to differentiate between CD and ulcerative colitis. Indeed, ASCA is detected in 55%-60% of children and adults with CD and only 5%-10% of controls with other gastrointestinal disorders. This finding pANCA highlights the relatively good specificity but poor sensitivity of ASCA as a marker

for CD. pANCA on the other hand is more specific to ulcerative colitis and the combination of a positive ASCA test with a negative pANCA test has a positive predictive value of 96% and a specificity of 97% for CD. 5. *Genetic studies*-In addition, some *NOD2/ CARD15* gene polymorphisms, particularly *L1007P* homozygosity, were found to be associated with gastroduodenal CD and with younger age at diagnosis. It is possible that these genes might also help to support the diagnosis in the atypical presentation of CD in the future. [2].

Differential Diagnosis

The differential diagnosis of the upper gastrointestinal tract endoscopic findings in Crohn's disease includes peptic ulcer disease, carcinoma, lymphoma, sarcoidosis, tuberculosis, eosinophilic gastroenteritis, Zollinger-Ellison syndrome, pancreatitis, and pancreatic cancer [4, 6].

The differential diagnosis includes corrosive gastritis due to ingestion of lye, gastric scirrhous carcinoma, Ménétrier's disease,. Pseudolymphoma, amyloidosis can also mimic Crohn's disease of the stomach [29]. Although Ménétrier's disease can involve the entire stomach and produce ulcérations, it does not cause transmural disease [29]. Malignant and infiltrative processes are to be ruled out by the histological findings.

Treatment

No controlled, prospective treatment studies have been reported for gastroduodenal Crohn's disease [4, 5].

1. *Medical treatment* - Most experts recommend intense acid suppression with a proton pump inhibitor. Peptic ulcer disease and *H. pylori* should be excluded and, if present, treated [4]. Occasionally this treatment is sufficient to allow healing of the gastroduodenal Crohn's disease as well. Most of the time, additional treatment must be provided for Crohn's disease of the small bowel and colon, which often coexist [3, 4]. Treatment should be based on symptom severity in individual patients [4]. Initial treatment for active gastric Crohn's disease often involves corticosteroids along with a proton pump

inhibitor [5, 7, 9, 36, 37]. Not all studies demonstrated corticosteroid-induced remission in active disease, however [10, 11, 34, 36-38]. 6-Mercaptopurine and azathioprine have been shown to maintain corticosteroid-induced remission and should be instituted early in the disease course [37-39]. Aminosalicylic acid compounds are generally not beneficial in upper gastrointestinal Crohn's disease and may aggravate symptoms [37]. The role of infliximab remains to be defined [2, 4, 6].

2. *Balloon dialation* - Strictures can complicate the course of gastroduodenal Crohn's disease. Short pyloric or duodenal strictures are ideal for endoscopic balloon dilation [4, 5]. Successful endoscopic dilation with a Rigiflex balloon (8 mm, Boston Scientific, Natick, Mass) or a Microvasive balloon (10 to 20 mm, Boston Scientific, Natick, Mass) has been described, with a risk of perforation of 1% to 2% [4, 40]. Often, repeated endoscopic dilation is required to completely treat strictures [41, 42]. In one series, 5 patients with obstructive gastroduodenal Crohn's disease were treated with endoscopic balloon dilation with an 18- to 20-mm balloon [40]. Each of the initial dilations was successful; 3 of the 5 patients had recurrent symptoms that required repeat dilations every 3 to 4 months [40]. All 5 patients avoided surgery during a mean follow-up interval of 4.2 years with concomitant use of either a proton pump inhibitor or histamine-2 receptor blocker [40]
3. *Surgical intervention* - One third of patients with gastroduodenal Crohn's disease does not respond to medical therapy alone and require surgery [43]. Additional indications for surgery include massive, persistent upper gastrointestinal hemorrhage, gastric outlet obstruction, and fistula or abscess formation [4, 5, 7, 10, 12, 44]. The most common indications for surgery are duodenal obstruction and refractory ulcer-type abdominal pain [6]. Before surgical therapy is initiated, patients should undergo upper gastrointestinal tract endoscopy, small bowel radiography, and colonoscopy for assessment of the extent of Crohn's disease to allow optimal surgical planning [6]. Surgical options in gastroduodenal Crohn's disease include bypass surgery with gastrojejunostomy (with or without vagotomy), commonly to bypass a duodenal stricture, gastroduodenostomy, duodenojejunostomy, and stricturoplasty [6, 7, 9]. Due to postvagotomy diarrhea and marginal ulcers after bypass surgery, gastrojejunostomy with highly selective vagotomy, preserving

autonomic innervation to the small bowel, should be regarded as the ideal surgical treatment of gastroduodenal Crohn's disease [43]. Gastric emptying may be delayed postoperatively in up to 24% of patients undergoing bypass surgery, but this complication may be seen in patients treated with stricturoplasty as well [6, 45, 46]. Other postoperative complications include anastomotic leak, enterocutaneous fistula, intraabdominal abscess, and stomal ulceration [47].

Conclusion

To conclude, Crohn's disease with isolated gastric involvement is an extremely unusual event in clinical practice. Endoscopic biopsy along with battery of laboratory tests is an effective tool to hit the correct diagnosis by excluding other causes of granulomatous gastritis. This prevents untoward mortality and /morbidity related to disease and treatment for the sake of accurate pathological diagnosis

References

[1] Ingle S B, Pujari G P, Patle YG, Nagoba BS. An unusual case of Crohn's disease with isolated gastric involvement. *J Crohns Colitis.* 2011;5:69–70. [PubMed]

[2] Sachin B Ingle, Chitra R Hinge, Sarita Dakhure , and Smita S Bhosale. Isolated gastric Crohn's disease. *World Journal of Clinical Cases.* May 16, 2013; 1(2): 71–73. Published online May 16, 2013. DOI: 10.12998/wjcc.v1.i2.71.

[3] Isaacs KL. Upper gastrointestinal tract endoscopy in inflammatory bowel disease. *Gastrointest Endosc Clin North Am* 2002;12:451–462.

[4] Burakoff R. Gastroduodenal Crohn's disease. In Bayless TM, Hanauer SB, eds. Advanced Therapy of Inflammatory Bowel Disease. Hamilton, Ontario: BC Decker, 2001:421–423.

[5] Banerjee S, Peppercorn MA. Inflammatory bowel disease. Medical therapy of specific clinical presentations. *Gastroenterol Clin North Am* 2002;31:185–202.

[6] Reynolds HL Jr, Stellato TA. Crohn's disease of the foregut. *Surg Clin North Am* 2001;81:117–135.

[7] Van Hogezand RA, Witte AM, Veenendaal RA, Wagtmans MJ, Lamers CB. Proximal Crohn's disease: review of the clinicopathologic features and therapy. *Inflamm Bowel Dis* 2001;7: 328–337.

[8] Sands BE. Crohn's disease. In Feldman M, Friedman LS, Sleisenger MH, eds. Sleisenger & Fordtran's Gastrointestinal and Liver Disease, 7th ed. Philadelphia:Saunders, 2002:2005–2038.

[9] Loftus EV Jr. Upper gastrointestinal tract Crohn's disease. *Clin Perspect Gastroenterol* 2002; 5: 188–191.

[10] Nugent FW, Richmond M, Park SK. Crohn's disease of the duodenum. *Gut* 1977;18: 115–120.

[11] Nugent FW, Roy MA. Duodenal Crohn's disease: an analysis of 89 cases. *Am J Gastroenterol* 1989;84 : 249–254.

[12] Wagtmans MJ, Verspaget HW, Lamers CB, van Hogezand RA. Clinical aspects of Crohn's disease of the upper gastrointestinal tract: a comparison with distal Crohn's disease. *Am J Gastroenterol* 1997;92 : 1467–1471.

[13] Bach JF. The effect of infections on susceptibility to autoimmune and allergic diseases. *N Engl J Med* 2002; 347: 911-920.

[14] Danese S, Sans M, Fiocchi C. Infl ammatory bowel disease: the role of environmental factors. *Autoimmun Rev* 2004; 3: 394-400.

[15] Lodes MJ, Cong Y, Elson CO, Mohamath R, Landers CJ, Targan SR, Fort M, Hershberg RM. Bacterial flagellin is a dominant antigen in Crohn disease. *J Clin Invest* 2004; 113: 1296-1306.

[16] Targan SR, Landers CJ, Yang H, Lodes MJ, Cong Y, Papadakis KA, Vasiliauskas E, Elson CO, Hershberg RM. Antibodies to CBir1 fl agellin defi ne a unique response that isassociated independently with complicated Crohn's disease. *Gastroenterology* 2005; 128: 2020-2028.

[17] Neurath MF, Weigmann B, Finotto S , Glickman J , Nieuwenhuis E, Iijima H, Mizoguchi A, Mizoguchi E, Mudter J, Galle PR, Bhan A, Autschbach F, Sullivan BM, Szabo SJ, Glimcher LH, Blumberg RS. The transcription factor T-bet regulates mucosal T cell activation in experimental colitis and Crohn's disease. *J Exp Med* 2002; 195: 1129-1143.

[18] Monteleone G, Biancone L, Marasco R, Morrone G, Marasco O, Luzza F, Pallone F. Interleukin 12 is expressed and actively released by Crohn's disease intestinal lamina propria mononuclear cells. *Gastroenterology* 1997; 112: 1169-1178.

[19] Pizarro TT, Michie MH, Bentz M, Woraratanadharm J, Smith MF Jr, Foley E, Moskaluk CA, Bickston SJ, Cominelli F. IL-18, a novel immunoregulatory cytokine, is up-regulated in Crohn's disease: expression and localization in intestinal mucosal cells. *J Immunol* 1999; 162: 6829-6835.
[20] Ina K, Itoh J, Fukushima K, Kusugami K, Yamaguchi T, Kyokane K, Imada A, Binion DG, Musso A, West GA, Dobrea GM, McCormick TS, Lapetina EG, Levine AD, Ottaway CA, Fiocchi C. Resistance of Crohn's disease T cells to multiple apoptotic signals is associated with a Bcl-2/Bax mucosal imbalance. *J Immunol* 1999; 163: 1081-1090.
[21] Sturm A, Leite AZ, Danese S, Krivacic KA, West GA, Mohr S, Jacobberger JW, Fiocchi C. Divergent cell cycle kinetics underlie the distinct functional capacity of mucosal T cells in Crohn's disease and ulcerative colitis. *Gut* 2004; 53: 1624-1631.
[22] Sakaguchi S. Naturally arising Foxp3-expressing CD25+CD4+ regulatory T cells in immunological tolerance to self and nonself. *Nat Immunol* 2005; 6: 345-352.
[23] Maul J, Loddenkemper C, Mundt P, Berg E, Giese T, Stallmach A, Zeitz M, Duchmann R. Peripheral and intestinal regulatory CD4+ CD25(high) T cells in inflammatory bowel disease. *Gastroenterology* 2005; 128: 1868-1878.
[24] Hart AL, Al-Hassi HO, Rigby RJ, Bell SJ, Emmanuel AV, Knight SC, Kamm MA, Stagg AJ. Characteristics of intestinal dendritic cells in infl ammatory bowel diseases. *Gastroenterology* 2005; 129: 50-65.
[25] Wehkamp J, Harder J, Weichenthal M, Schwab M, Schaffeler E, Schlee M, Herrlinger KR, Stallmach A, Noack F, Fritz P, Schroder JM, Bevins CL, Fellermann K, Stange EF. NOD2 (CARD15) mutations in Crohn‘s disease are associated with diminished mucosal alpha-defensin expression. *Gut* 2004; 53:1658-1664.
[26] Rogler G. Update in inflammatory bowel disease pathogenesis. *Curr Opin Gastroenterol* 2004; 20: 311-317.
[27] Rutgeerts P, Onette E, Vantrappen G, Geboes K, Broeckaert L, Talloen L.Crohn’s disease of the stomach and duodenum: a clinical study with emphasis on the value of endoscopy and endoscopic biopsies. *Endoscopy* 1980;12:288–294.
[28] Levine MS. Crohn’s disease of the upper gastrointestinal tract. *Radiol Clin North Am* 1987;25:79–91.
[29] Cary ER, Tremaine WJ, Banks PM, Nagorney DM. Isolated Crohn’s disease of the stomach. *Mayo Clin Proc* 1989;64:776–779.

[30] Danzi JT, Farmer RG, Sullivan BH Jr, Rankin GB. Endoscopic features of gastroduodenal Crohn's disease. *Gastroenterology* 1976;70:9–13.

[31] Alcantara M, Rodriguez R, Potenciano JL, Carrobles JL, Munoz C, Gomez R. Endoscopic and bioptic findings in the upper gastrointestinal tract in patients with Crohn's disease. *Endoscopy* 1993;25:282–286.

[32] Fenoglio-Preiser CM, Noffsinger AE, Stemmermann GN, Lantz PE, Listrom MB, Rilke FO. The non neoplastic stomach. In Gastrointestinal Pathology, 2nd ed. Philadelphia: *Lippincott-Raven*, 1999:153–236.

[33] Halme L, Karkkainen P, Rautelin H, Kosunen TU, Sipponen P. High frequency of helicobacter negative gastritis in patients with Crohn's disease. *Gut* 1996;38:379–383.

[34] Oberhuber G, Puspok A, Oesterreicher C, Novacek G, Zauner C, Burghuber M, Vogelsang H, Potzi R, Stolte M, Wrba F. Focally enhanced gastritis: a frequent type of gastritis in patients with Crohn's disease. *Gastroenterology* 1997;112:698–706.

[35] Parente F, Cucino C, Bollani S, Imbesi V, Maconi G, Bonetto S, Vago L, Porro GB. Focal gastric inflammatory infiltrates in inflammatory bowel diseases: prevalence, immunohistochemical characteristics, and diagnostic role. *Am J Gastroenterol* 2000;95:705–711.

[36] Miehsler W, Puspok A, Oberhuber T, Vogelsang H. Impact of different therapeutic regimens on the outcome of patients with Crohn's disease of the upper gastrointestinal tract. *Inflamm Bowel Dis* 2001;7: 99–105.

[37] Valori RM, Cockel R. Omeprazole for duodenal ulceration in Crohn's disease. *BMJ* 1990; 300:438–439.

[38] Griffiths AM, Alemayehu E, Sherman P. Clinical features of gastroduodenal Crohn's disease in adolescents. *J Pediatr Gastroenterol Nutr* 1989;8:166 – 171.

[39] Korelitz BI, Adler DJ, Mendelsohn RA, Sacknoff AL. Long-term experience with 6-mercaptopurine in the treatment of Crohn's disease. *Am J Gastroenterol* 1993;88:1198–1205.

[40] Matsui T, Hatakeyama S, Ikeda K, Yao T, Takenaka K, Sakurai T. Longterm outcome of endoscopic balloon dilation in obstructive gastroduodenal Crohn's disease. *Endoscopy* 1997;29:640–645.

[41] Dancygier H, Frick B. Crohn's disease of the upper gastrointestinal tract. *Endoscopy* 1992;24:555–558.

[42] Murthy UK. Repeated hydrostatic balloon dilation in obstructive gastroduodenal Crohn's disease. *Gastrointest Endosc* 1991;37:484–485.

[43] Marcello PW, Schoetz DJ Jr. Gastroduodenal Crohn's disease: surgical management. In Bayless TM, Hanauer SB, eds. Advanced Therapy of

Inflammatory Bowel Disease. Hamilton, Ontario: BC Decker, 2001:461–463.

[44] Murray JJ, Schoetz DJ Jr, Nugent FW, Coller JA, Veidenheimer MC. Surgical management of Crohn's disease involving the duodenum. *Am J Surg* 1984;147:58–65.

[45] Worsey MJ, Hull T, Ryland L, Fazio V. Strictureplasty is an effective option in the operative management of duodenal Crohn's disease. *Dis Colon Rectum* 1999;42:596–600.

[46] Yamamoto T, Bain IM, Connolly AB, Allan RN, Keighley MR. Outcome of strictureplasty for duodenal Crohn's disease. *Br J Surg* 1999;86:259–262.

[47] Yamamoto T, Allan RN, Keighley MR. An audit of gastroduodenal Crohn disease: clinicopathologic features and management. *Scand J Gastroenterol* 1999;34:1019–1024.

Chapter 6

Melanosis coli

Introduction

Melanosis coli, also *pseudomelanosis coli*, is a disorder of pigmentation of the wall of the colon, often identified at the time of colonoscopy. It is benign, and may have no significant correlation with disease. The brown pigment is lipofuscin in macrophages, not melanin.

Etiology

The most common cause of *melanosis coli* is the extended use of laxatives, and commonly anthraquinone containing laxatives such as Senna and other plant glycosides. [1] The anthranoid laxatives pass through the gastrointestinal tract unabsorbed until they reach the large intestine, where they are changed into their active forms. The resulting active compounds cause damage to the cells in the lining of the intestine and leads to apoptosis (a form of cell death). The damaged (apoptotic) cells appear as darkly pigmented bodies that may be taken up by scavenger cells known as macrophages. When enough cells have been damaged, the characteristic pigmentation of the bowel wall develops. The condition can develop after just a few months of laxative use. [2]

However, other causes are identified, including an increase in colonic epithelial apoptosis. [3] Endoscopically, the mucosa may show a brownish discoloration in a moire pattern.

Histologic Appearance

On biopsy, *melanosis coli* shows characteristic pigment-laden macrophages within the mucosa (Figure 1) on PAS staining. [4]

The histologic differential diagnosis of mucosal pigmentation is: lipofuscin (melanosis coli), hemosiderin-laden macrophages, and melanin (rare).

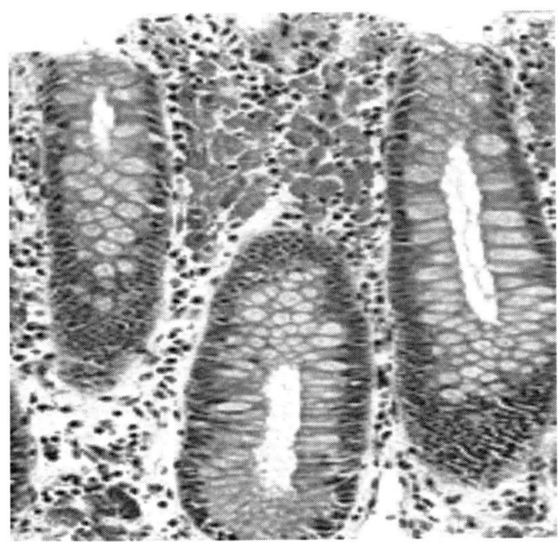

Figure 1. Showing pigment-laden macrophages within the mucosa.

Prognosis

No adverse effects or consequences of melanosis coli have been identified. [4]

Relation to True Melanoses

The condition is unrelated to true melanoses, such as Peutz-Jeghers syndrome and smoker's melanosis. [5]

Peutz-Jegher syndrome causes pigmentation of the skin and mucous surfaces with melanin, and polyps in the digestive tract.

Non-colonic Pseudomelanoses

Pseudomelanoses of other parts of the gastrointestinal tract have also been reported, and are of unclear relevance. [6]

Patients with colostomies can have melanosis involving the stoma, which is also of no significance. [7]

References

[1] Müller-Lissner, SA. (Oct 1993). "Adverse effects of laxatives: fact and fiction." *Pharmacology* 47 (Suppl 1): 138–45. doi:10.1159/000139853. PMID 8234421.

[2] http://www.medicinenet.com/melanosis_coli/page2.htm

[3] Byers, R.J.; Marsh, P.; Parkinson, D.; Haboubi, N.Y (October 2003). "Melanosis coli are associated with an increase in colonic epithelial apoptosis and not with laxative use". *Histopathology* 30 (2): 160–164. doi:10.1046/j.1365-2559.1997.d01-574.x. PMID 9067741.

[4] Wittoesch, JH.; Jackman, RJ.; McDonald, JR. "Melanosis coli: general review and a study of 887 cases." *Dis Colon Rectum* 1 (3): 172–80. PMID 13537819.

[5] Vellappally, S.; Fiala, Z.; Smejkalová, J.; Jacob, V.; Somanathan, R. (2007). "Smoking related systemic and oral diseases." *Acta Medica* (Hradec Kralove) 50 (3): 161–6. PMID 18254267.

[6] Ghadially, FN.; Walley, VM. (Sep 1994). "Melanoses of the gastrointestinal tract." *Histopathology* 25 (3): 197–207. doi:10.1111/j.1365-2559.1994.tb01319.x. PMID 7821887.

[7] Fleischer, I.; Bryant, D. (May 1995). "Melanosis coli or mucosa ischemia? A case report." *Ostomy Wound Manage* 41 (4): 44, 46–7. PMID 7598783.

Index

E

F

G

H

I

K

L

Q

R

S